D0891584

THE **MICROBIOME DIET**

Also by Raphael Kellman, MD

Gut Reactions

Matrix Healing

THE
MICROBIOME DIET

*The Scientifically Proven Way to Restore Your Gut Health
and Achieve Permanent Weight Loss*

By Raphael Kellman, MD

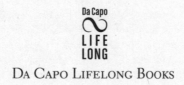

DA CAPO LIFELONG BOOKS

Designed by Linda Mark
Set in 12 point Electra LT Std by the Perseus Books Group

Library of Congress Cataloging-in-Publication Data
Kellman, Raphael, 1960–
   The microbiome diet : the scientifically proven way to restore your gut health
and achieve permanent weight loss / by Raphael Kellman, MD.—First Da Capo
Press edition.
      pages cm
   Includes index.
    ISBN 978-0-7382-1765-9 (hardback)—ISBN 978-0-7382-1766-6 (e-book)
1. Weight loss—Popular works. 2. Metabolism—Popular works. 3. Human
body—Microbiology. I. Title.
   RM222.2.K4479 2014
   613.2'5—dc23

                                                                        2014006125

ISBN 978-0-7382-1820-5 (international edition)

First Da Capo Press edition 2014
Published by Da Capo Press
A Member of the Perseus Books Group
www.dacapopress.com

Note: The information in this book is true and complete to the best of our
knowledge. This book is intended only as an informative guide for those
wishing to know more about health issues. In no way is this book intended
to replace, countermand, or conflict with the advice given to you by your
own physician. The ultimate decision concerning care should be made
between you and your doctor. We strongly recommend you follow his or
her advice. Information in this book is general and is offered with no
guarantees on the part of the authors or Da Capo Press. The authors and
publisher disclaim all liability in connection with the use of this book.

Da Capo Press books are available at special discounts for bulk purchases
in the U.S. by corporations, institutions, and other organizations. For more
information, please contact the Special Markets Department at the Perseus
Books Group, 2300 Chestnut Street, Suite 200, Philadelphia, PA, 19103, or
call (800) 810-4145, ext. 5000, or e-mail special.markets@perseusbooks.com.

10 9 8 7 6 5 4 3 2 1

To my beautiful wife, Chasya, whom I love deeply.
I am so grateful that we share the same loving worldview.

CONTENTS

PART I

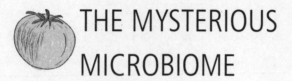 THE MYSTERIOUS
MICROBIOME

one

THE WORLD WITHIN YOUR GUT

IF I EVER MET ANYONE WHO SEEMED TO DEFY ALL CONVENTIONAL RULES for weight loss, it was Robert.

Robert just could not manage to lose weight.

He was a middle-aged man who was my patient about eight years ago. I was treating him for multiple health problems—heart disease, high blood pressure, high levels of insulin, and a blood sugar reading that I was very concerned about. But I knew that all of these issues would greatly improve—and perhaps even disappear—if we could just get Robert down to a healthy weight.

Before he had become my patient Robert had been on every diet in the book. Atkins, the Zone, low-carb, low-fat—you name it, Robert had tried it. But to his great frustration, none of these diets ever worked for him. He would starve himself for weeks, trying to stick to the rules he had been given, only to find that he could barely lose five pounds. Then, the moment he broke the diet even a little bit—a single forbidden baked potato when he took a client to a steakhouse, splitting a piece of chocolate cake with his wife on their anniversary—he would gain back even the little weight he had lost. By the time he came to see me, Robert had simply given up.

So for most of the time I had been treating him Robert was nearly fifty pounds above his ideal weight. He drank, he smoked, he ate all the wrong things, and I simply could not get him to adopt a healthy lifestyle.

"What's the use, Doc?" he would always ask me. "No matter what I do, the weight doesn't come off. So why bother trying?"

Now he was in the hospital with pneumonia. When I thought about the potential effect that might have on his weight, my heart sank. Robert had had previous hospital stays for different ailments, and he had always emerged five to seven pounds heavier. The combination of starchy hospital food and lack of movement exacerbated his tendency to gain weight, and I always dreaded the aftereffects of his prolonged periods of bed rest.

This time, however, I was treating Robert with a course of antibiotics. To counter the effects of the antibiotics I was also treating him with *probiotics*. Antibiotics kill the bacteria that make us sick, but they also kill the healthy bacteria that live throughout our bodies, especially in our intestinal tract. Probiotics counter the destruction that antibiotics cause—and sometimes, as we shall see, they have even more powerful effects.

I had also prescribed *prebiotics* for Robert. Prebiotics are foods and supplements that nourish healthy bacteria. Whereas probiotics help to replace the healthy bacteria that have been destroyed, prebiotics help to support the healthy bacteria that still remain.

So this time, instead of gaining weight, Robert *lost* seven pounds in two weeks—without making any effort at all. Why?

Trying to solve this mystery led me on a journey I never expected: the discovery of a new approach to diet and health that transformed my own understanding of weight loss and one that I hope will transform yours too. I believe that this book will challenge everything you know about the causes of obesity—and about the kind of diet that can successfully overcome it.

Thanks to Robert, I was able to develop a diet that benefited dozens of my patients, helping them lose weight quickly and to keep it off forever.

Patients who followed this new approach were able to lose pounds, inches, and body fat, especially around the stomach, waist, and abdomen.

They found that after years of struggling to lose those stubborn pounds they could never get rid of, all of a sudden the weight was coming off by itself.

They discovered that within a few days they began to lose their cravings for sugar, bread, baked goods, and other "forbidden foods," such as macaroni and cheese, pizza, and ice cream, and within a few weeks those cravings were gone completely. For the first time they could remember they no longer felt like a prisoner of their own appetites, forever longing for foods they knew were not good for their health.

Best of all, once my patients had spent a few weeks on this diet they were able to drop to only 90 percent compliance. After a few more weeks on this diet they were able to maintain only 70 percent compliance—*all while remaining at their healthy weight!* My new approach to weight loss had enabled my patients to reset and reboot their sluggish metabolism so they could periodically indulge in an occasional rich food or sweet dessert without fear of developing the old cravings—or gaining back the old weight. And unlike the vast majority of dieters, who tend to regain all the old weight and more, the people on *this* diet continued to maintain a healthy weight for years.

What is the secret to this extraordinarily successful weight loss plan? What mystery had my patient Robert unlocked for me on his "accidental diet"? The answer lies in the *microbiome,* the mysterious but oh-so-important world that each of us holds within.

THE MICROBIOME: KEY WEIGHT LOSS FACTS

- 90 percent of the cells within your body are not human—they are microbes and bacteria known as the *microbiome*.
- The microbiome is the key to revving up your metabolism and losing weight.
- You don't have to count calories, fats, or carbs to lose weight; you just have to avoid the foods that hurt your microbiome and eat the foods that support it.
- After seven weeks you can maintain only 70 percent compliance, indulging in other foods up to 30 percent of the time.

THE MICROBIOME: A WEIGHT LOSS BREAKTHROUGH

What if I told you that 90 percent of the cells within your body are *not human*?

And what if I told you that this nonhuman 90 percent—an entire separate ecology within your own body—is the key to losing weight and keeping it off?

A series of scientific breakthroughs over the last few years has revealed that the key to fast, permanent weight loss is the *microbiome*—the trillions of tiny bacteria living within our intestines.

While millions of people have been struggling with all kinds of diets—and either failing to lose weight or gaining back all the weight they lost—a whole new paradigm has begun to emerge.

Cutting-edge science has shown that the microbiome is the secret to healthy, dramatic weight loss as well as significant improvements to your overall health, mood, energy, and mental function. Research reveals that when the microbiome goes out of balance, people often gain weight, even when they haven't changed their diet or exercise. An imbalanced microbiome often dooms just about any diet to failure. When the microbiome is balanced, however, people often lose weight, even when they don't make any other changes.

These microscopic organisms regulate the way calories are extracted from your food. They produce vital nutrients and help regulate your immune system. They exert enormous influence over your hormones, your appetite, your cravings, and even your genes. They also have a huge impact on your *neurotransmitters*, the brain chemicals that govern your mood, energy levels, and mental functioning.

Most important of all, however, is the way the microbiome affects your *metabolism*. When your metabolism is revved up and working at top speed, you lose weight and keep it off, effortlessly maintaining a healthy weight. When your metabolism is sluggish and cued to retain body fat, you will gain weight and hold onto those extra pounds even if you cut way back on the calories and ramp up the exercise.

Metabolism is the key to weight loss. And the microbiome is the key to metabolism.

The microbiome was the reason Robert had suddenly lost weight, effortlessly, after years of unsuccessful dieting. The microbiome was the reason Robert no longer craved sweets and starches, fried foods and fatty meats, potato chips and cheesecake. The microbiome was the reason Robert no longer felt hungry all the time and why he finally felt satisfied after he ate. Best of all, the microbiome was the reason Robert could occasionally enjoy that baked potato or chocolate cake—as much as 30 percent of the time.

Robert's experience—and the knowledge I sought as a result—convinced me that supporting and balancing the microbiome can be the basis for a fast, effective, and long-lasting approach to weight loss. Supporting the microbiome might even be the solution to the worldwide obesity epidemic. So let's take a closer look at this mysterious but crucial portion of your anatomy.

WHAT IS THE MICROBIOME?

The microbiome is a miniature world made up of trillions of microscopic, nonhuman organisms that flourish within your gastrointestinal tract. These intestinal organisms—bacteria—digest your food, govern your appetite, control your metabolism, orchestrate your immune system, influence your mood, and even help determine how your genes are expressed. They have a major impact on whether your heart is healthy, whether your bones develop properly, and whether your brain feels sharp and clear or fuzzy and unfocused. They sustain the gastrointestinal tract so your food is properly digested and you get all the nourishment you need. They produce crucial vitamins and other nutrients. They even manufacture natural antibiotics.

Most amazing of all, these nonhuman organisms make up a whopping 90 percent of your cells!

Think about that for a moment. The vast majority of the cells within your body are *not human*. Within your intestinal tract lies a whole separate ecology that is inextricably involved with yours. When these microscopic organisms flourish, you flourish. When they struggle, you struggle. When they crave sugar, so do you. And when they operate at peak efficiency, so does your metabolism.

That is why balancing your microbiome is the key to eliminating food cravings.

It is the key to eliminating symptoms that you might never even have connected to your weight and the way you eat, such as fatigue, anxiety, depression, brain fog, headaches, acne, eczema, congestion, frequent colds and infections, joint pain, and muscle pain.

Balancing your microbiome is also the key to preventing and even reversing major illnesses, including diabetes, heart disease, metabolic syndrome, autoimmune disorders, autism, and other developmental disorders

I knew about the microbiome when I began treating Robert, but I didn't know about its connection to weight loss. I had prescribed those probiotics and prebiotics for Robert as part of my effort to improve his intestinal health. The "invader" bacteria causing Robert's pneumonia had also caused Robert's microbial system to become even more imbalanced. The antibiotics I had prescribed to kill off the bad bacteria would help cure the pneumonia, while the probiotics and prebiotics I gave him helped Robert rebalance his inner ecology. As a result, Robert's pneumonia was cured, and at the same time he lost weight, without even trying, simply because his microbial health had been restored.

ANTIBIOTICS, PROBIOTICS, AND PREBIOTICS

Antibiotics can have a near-miraculous effect on many diseases, but they can also wreak havoc with the microbiome, as we shall see, creating multiple health problems and a greatly increased risk for weight gain. If you need to take antibiotics, be sure to also follow my Microbiome Diet recommendations for probiotics and prebiotics, on page 79. *Probiotics* are microscopic organisms that will replenish your microbiome. *Prebiotics* are foods and supplements that nourish the organisms already in your microbiome.

In fact, by themselves antibiotics don't lead to weight loss but, instead, to weight gain—and for the same reason. Antibiotics are designed to kill the unhealthy bacteria within our bodies, but often, like a spray of gunfire, they wipe out innocent bystanders as well, destroying our good bacteria and throwing our microbiome out of balance. The underlying principle is clear:

> **Our metabolism, weight, and overall
> health depend on the balance of microbial
> life within our gastrointestinal tract.**

THE MICROBIOME AND YOUR HEALTH

Perhaps it's because I have a four-year-old daughter, but when I imagine the microbiome I think of that old Dr. Seuss story *Horton Hears a Who*. If you recall, Horton the elephant had enormous ears that enabled him to hear tiny sounds that others missed. As a result, he was able to detect an entire civilization of microscopic organisms, called Whoville, situated on a minuscule speck of dust.

Because Horton's neighbors could not perceive that microscopic world, they were skeptical and even angry when Horton tried to get them to acknowledge, respect, and protect it. In fact, they were ready to destroy the entire community of Whoville simply because they could not see it. "A person's a person, no matter how small," Horton kept repeating, but his respect for the miniature world he had discovered angered his neighbors even more.

Just as Horton's neighbors could not perceive the tiny residents of "Whoville," so do most of us remain unaware of the microscopic world within us. And just as Horton's neighbors did not understand their responsibility for preserving that unseen community, so do most of us fail to understand our own responsibility for supporting our microbiome—with disastrous results for our weight, our metabolism, and our health.

I know it sounds like the stuff of fantasy, but we really do contain within our bodies an entire ecology of nonhuman organisms—bacterial flora and fauna living inside us in a symbiotic relationship. The ecology that lives within our intestines is dependent on us. And we, likewise, depend on it. Healing this ecology and keeping it in balance is the key to our overall health.

Scientists have known about the microbiome for a long time, but only recently have we begun to understand its importance. In 2008 the National Institutes of Health began a project to map the microbiome, triggering an enormous amount of exciting research. Cutting-edge studies reveal that in addition to helping us resist disease, depression, and anxiety, the microbiome is crucial to our metabolism, our hunger, our eating patterns, and our weight.

We used to think that all microbes were unhealthy bacteria determined to infect us with deadly diseases. Now we are beginning to understand that most microbes are actually helpful to us, performing so many important functions that, without them, we could not survive.

When we eat the foods that keep this inner world in balance, our metabolism runs at peak efficiency. Our bodies almost effortlessly maintain their ideal weight. We feel hungry only when we really need more food, and we feel full and satisfied when we have had enough. We lose the body fat that distorts our shape, regaining our healthy waistlines and relatively flat abdomens. We also feel more vital and energized than ever before; dispel our brain fog, sleep problems, depression, and anxiety; and develop healthy, glowing skin and hair. This is why I say that balancing our microbiome is the key to optimum weight and health.

By contrast, when we consume foods or medicines that throw this inner world out of balance, we put ourselves at risk for a host of diseases, from skin rashes to cancer. We feel tired, anxious, grouchy, depressed, or just plain "not ourselves." We feel hungry much of the time—perhaps even all the time—regardless of whether we need the food. And, ultimately, we accumulate body fat, especially around the abdomen, gaining weight that is virtually impossible to lose and even harder to keep off.

THE FORGOTTEN ORGAN

Most of us tend to think of ourselves as separate, autonomous beings whose growth and development depend entirely on ourselves. But in fact, our health, our weight, and our very survival are inextricably dependent on our microbiome.

As soon as we pass through the birth canal we begin to become 90 percent microbe. The moment we come into this world we start the process of acquiring the trillions of bacteria that we need to achieve optimal health. In fact, the microbiome is so important to our survival that it has been dubbed "the forgotten organ."

One of the first bacteria we encounter is called *Lactobacillus johnsonii*, a microscopic creature we acquire in the birth canal. This microbe digests milk and, therefore, helps us metabolize our mother's breast milk.

Significantly, our mother's milk itself contains oligosaccharides, a type of prebiotic that feeds our microbiome. As infants, we cannot digest this substance, but our microbes can. How important must our microbiome be to our survival if mother's milk itself nourishes this nonhuman but crucial portion of our anatomy?

Scientists are just beginning to realize the importance of the microbes acquired during that trip down the birth canal, because babies who don't have that initial access to their mother's microbiome—that is, babies who are delivered by Caesarean section—are often prey

YEAST INFECTIONS AND UTIS

If you're prone to frequent infections in the vaginal area, an unbalanced microbiome might be the cause. Following the Microbiome Diet will help rebalance your microbiome and prevent further infections.

to a number of immune-related disorders, such as asthma, allergies, celiac disease, and skin infections. Some studies suggest that babies born by C-section also face a higher risk of Type 1 diabetes and obesity—a further connection between the microbiome, metabolism, and weight. Likewise, many researchers now believe that when children are given antibiotics, which can devastate the microbiome, they face a higher risk of allergy-related diseases, inflammatory bowel syndrome, and, again, obesity.

Although each microbe is small, those trillions of tiny organisms add up to a weight of about three pounds—coincidentally, what your brain weighs as well. Your "forgotten organ" occupies your digestive system, mouth, nasal passages, and lungs as well as living on your skin and in your brain. If you're a woman, as we just saw, the microbiome also inhabits your vaginal canal. A healthy microbiome supports your health in each region, whereas an out-of-balance microbiome leaves you prone to infection, imbalance, and distress.

Scientists have come to believe that the more diverse your microbiome—the more species it contains—the healthier you are likely to be *and* the better you will be able to control unwanted weight gain. So far, researchers have identified about ten thousand species of bacteria that potentially occupy the human microbiome, but each person's microbiome has its own unique combination. Even identical twins have been shown to have individual microbiomes.

At the same time, we tend to acquire bacteria from the people we live and work with and perhaps even from casual contacts in a crowded street or packed room. This is possible because your microbiome is extremely dynamic, able to change composition within twenty-four hours in response to stress, antibiotics, and illness and able to change within a few weeks or even days in response to diet, supplements, and exercise.

In fact, many scientists are concerned about the ways in which our microbiomes are changing, because those of us in the developed world seem to be losing microbial diversity with every generation. Those of us in the developed world tend to be treated with antibiotics frequently and to have relatively little contact with plants, animals, and soil. In addition, the Western diet includes a high proportion of refined foods, which also tends to kill off certain bacteria. As a result, our microbiomes tend to contain far fewer microbial species than people who grow up in developing nations. According to some scientists, the microbial diversity of developing nations is the reason for their lower rates of allergy and asthma: Diverse microbiomes are better at keeping the immune system in balance. To help respond to the various bacteria that it will encounter throughout your life, your immune system must be introduced to a wide variety of microbes.

Many scientists also believe that low microbial diversity correlates with weight gain. Some have even argued that the destruction of the microbiome is a prime mover behind the obesity epidemic. Martin J. Blaser, chair of the Department of Medicine and a professor of microbiology at the New York University School of Medicine, does not believe that bad eating habits are enough to cause our rapid and widespread explosion of obesity, and he's tried to prove this by creating his own mini-obesity epidemic among the mice in his laboratory simply by administering small but steady doses of antibiotics. The antibiotics kill off many of the mice's microbes, and the mice have gained enormous amounts of weight. Blaser believes a similar destruction of microbial diversity might help explain the worldwide obesity epidemic.

Other studies back up Blaser's hypothesis, including one reported in the August 29, 2013, issue of *Nature*. The Pan European Meta HIT Consortium studied nearly three hundred Danish volunteers, both lean and obese, whom it examined over the course of nine years. Researchers measured the bacterial genes found in the volunteers' stool along with weight gain and other markers of metabolic health, such as blood pressure, blood sugar levels, insulin levels, and inflammation, all of which can set you up for both weight gain and disorders like heart disease and diabetes.

And, indeed, the study discovered that for the volunteers who were already obese, a relatively low diversity in the microbiome correlated with significant weight gain over the course of nine years. Generally, low diversity correlated with higher inflammation, greater insulin resistance, and other danger signs of metabolic disorder.

WHY WE NEED THE "FORGOTTEN ORGAN"

I know it's challenging to wrap your mind around the idea that there is a whole other ecology within your body, an ecology that is not human but nevertheless an essential part of you as well as a crucial aspect of your health.

And yet it's true. The health of your microbiome determines the quality of your health, and without your microbiome you couldn't survive. In fact, without your microbiome you would no longer be *you*, just as you would no longer be you without your brain or your heart.

A balanced microbiome regulates your immune system, three-quarters of which is located within your intestines. It nourishes and sustains your gastrointestinal tract. It produces crucial vitamins and nutrients, including various B vitamins and vitamin K. It lays the groundwork for optimal mood and brain function by influencing the production of your *neurotransmitters*, the hormones and biochemicals your brain needs to process thought and emotion. And it keeps you at your ideal weight by helping you digest your food, maintain an appropriate appetite, regulating the calories that enter your system, and keeping your metabolism working at optimal speed.

Every human and animal on the planet has its own unique microbiome. But as scientists have become interested in this "forgotten organ," they wondered what might happen to animals who actually were raised without one. So they began breeding germ-free mice in sterile laboratory conditions to learn what happens when an animal is 100 percent itself instead of 90 percent microbe.

The results were startling. In the eloquent words of science journalist Moises Velasquez-Manoff, writing in *Mother Jones* in April 2013,

> Animals raised without microbes essentially lack a functioning immune system. Entire repertoires of white blood cells remain dormant; their intestines don't develop the proper creases and crypts; their hearts are shrunken; genes in the brain that should be in the "off" position remain stuck "on." Without their microbes, animals aren't really "normal."

In other words, our "forgotten organ" is a crucial aspect of our health and even our identity, from birth to death. And, as Robert and hundreds of my other patients have found, protecting and supporting this inner ecology is the fastest and most reliable route to losing unhealthy weight and permanently keeping it off.

THE MICROBIOME AND YOUR SECOND GENOME

The Human Genome Project was begun in 1990, an ambitious attempt to map the genes that make us human. Scientists involved in the project hoped that by better understanding our own DNA we would be able to unlock the genetic basis for a wide variety of illnesses, from allergies to cancer, and that this greater understanding would open up new possibilities for healing.

I too am excited about the new frontier of genetic medicine. But I am even more excited when I consider that each of us contains a *second* genome: the genetic material of the microbiome. And this second genome is in many ways even more powerful than the first.

After all, you come into the world with only about twenty-two thousand human genes. But as you acquire your microbiome, you incorporate into your body another 3.3 million genes—a ratio of about 150:1. As Velasquez-Manoff says, comparing the second genome to the first, "Think of it as a hulking instruction manual compared to a single page to-do list."

Our own genes change slowly, from generation to generation. But the life span of a microbe is only about twenty minutes. This means that your microbiome's genetic composition can change rapidly—so rapidly that within twenty-four hours you can completely imbalance your microbiome in response to stress, antibiotics, or major illness. Conversely, within just a few weeks you can begin to rebalance your microbiome through a healthy diet. This gives us tremendous plasticity—and tremendous control over our health, appetite, weight, and metabolism.

Not only does the microbiome have a tremendous impact on us via *their* genes, but they also have a huge impact on *our* genes. The ability to modify a gene's expression—to turn a gene on or off or to turn its volume up or down—is known as *epigenetics*, and it is one of the most exciting new frontiers in science and medicine. Rather than viewing your genes as fixed entities—inherited "givens" that determine your life—you can see them as a dynamic set of relationships that can be modified profoundly by what you eat, the nutrients and supplements you take, how well you sleep, and how you handle stress. In other words, you are not a slave to your genes. Other environmental factors come into play as well—and so does your second genome.

To illustrate how epigenetics works, let me offer an example. Many of us have a genetic predisposition to diabetes. A number of different genes are involved in this tendency, and they all must interact in a particular way to produce the disease. However, a diet high in sugar and starches can turn these genes on, and a healthy diet can turn them off. The genes themselves don't change, but their *expression* does.

Our genes can also predispose us to weight gain. Like diabetes, a number of genes are involved in this type of metabolism as well as several complicated interactions. However, that genetic inheritance can also be turned on or off. An unbalanced microbiome can activate a predisposition to obesity, and a healthy microbiome can turn those genes down or even off. So the genetic makeup of our microbiome determines how our "forgotten organ" will affect our genes.

The reverse is also true. Those of us with genes predisposed to a healthy weight can nonetheless become obese if stress, diet, lifestyle, or exposure to toxins undermines our microbiome. Genes tell a very important part of our story—but only one part.

When work began on the Human Genome Project many scientists believed our genes would offer us the ultimate answer to the riddle of human individuality. They thought perhaps our genes would explain the differences that make each of us unique.

What they found, however, was that all of us humans share around 99.9 percent of the same human DNA. The genetic differences between us are incredibly tiny compared to everything we have in common.

Conversely, no two people, including identical twins, share the same microbiome. Given that the genes of our microbiome outnumber ours by a factor of 150 to 1, perhaps *that* is where our diversity and uniqueness really lie. It seems our health—and perhaps even our biological destiny—has more to do with our second genome than our first.

When we consider how vital the microbiome is to our survival, how intricately involved it is with our immune system, metabolism, and weight, we begin to truly understand the concept of *symbiosis*, of living together. Because microbes were present as we evolved, our genes did not need to encode all of our vital information. Our bodies did not require preprogrammed instruction for every task involved in digestion, immunity, thought, or emotion; rather, we evolved as *interdependent* on microbial life, relying on our microbiome to perform tasks our brains and bodies cannot perform alone. In this light, evolution is not a matter of "survival of the fittest" but rather "survival of the wholest"!

This insight is particularly relevant when it comes to weight loss. Your microbiome harvests your calories, extracts crucial vitamins, helps you digest your food, decides whether you feel hungry or full, and regulates your metabolism to determine whether you store fat or burn it. You literally cannot perform those functions by yourself. To achieve your ideal appetite, metabolism, and weight, you need the help of your microbiome.

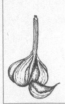

STOP COUNTING CALORIES!

As you will see when you begin the Microbiome Diet, on this program you don't count calories. Yet the calorie-counting model is so persistent among dieters that many of my patients can't quite believe I want them to stop thinking in those terms. Years of dieting have taught them that their weight is the result of how many calories they consume minus how many calories they burn. It's all about willpower: How well can they resist the seductive high-calorie treats that seem to beckon at every turn?

But I have news for you: your microbiome is stronger and smarter than you are. An imbalanced microbiome will overpower you with cravings for sugar and unhealthy fats, slowing down your metabolism and increasing your appetite. Conversely, a balanced microbiome will lead you to crave healthy foods, feel hungry and full at the right times, and, most important, rev up your metabolism and cause you to burn fat instead of storing it. Listen to a healthy microbiome and you'll never have to rely on willpower again.

Here's how I know that counting calories is the fastest road to a dead-end diet. In the developed world most of us consume far more calories than we actually need. However, *we don't gain weight in proportion to those calories.*

Consider a pound of human body fat. It contains roughly thirty-five hundred calories, which means that if you consumed just five hundred extra calories each day, you should gain a pound each week,

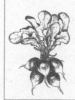

Yang-Xin Fu, MD, PhD, is a professor of pathology at the University of Chicago School of Medicine. In an August 2012 article in the journal *Nature Immunology* he argued that weight gain was not a simple matter of caloric overload but rather an interplay between intestinal microbes and the immune system, stating, "Diet-induced obesity depends not just on calories ingested, but also on the host's microbiome."

right? To put it in perspective, five hundred calories is half a bag of movie popcorn, a bagel with a big schmear of cream cheese, or two glasses of wine and a few slices of cheese.

Most of us do eat about that many extra calories each day. But few of us gain a pound a week, and some of us don't gain any weight at all.

Likewise, exercise is a huge support for a healthy weight, but you can't really detect that support by counting calories. A twenty-minute jog, for example, burns fewer than three hundred calories. That's not enough to account for significant weight loss. If we want to understand what causes us to lose or gain weight, we have to look further.

DON'T COUNT FATS OR CARBS EITHER

Clearly the "calories in–calories out" model simply doesn't work. So what about the *kind* of calories you consume? Consider this study by Walter Willett, MD, the highly respected professor at the Harvard School of Public Health.

Dr. Willett put eighteen hundred men and fifteen hundred women on three different types of diets for twelve weeks. Two groups ate the exact same amount of calories, but one group followed a low-fat diet while the other group followed a low-carb diet. The third group also followed a low-carb diet but with an extra three hundred calories.

Three months later the results were in. The low-fat group lost an average of seventeen pounds. Its low-carb counterpart lost a lot more weight, an average of twenty-three pounds. But the low-carb group that had consumed *more* calories than the low-fat group also lost more weight, an average of twenty pounds. In other words, you can lose more weight by cutting back more on carbs than on fat, even when you consume more calories!

Likewise, Dr. David Ludwig, a professor of nutrition at the Harvard School of Public Health, devised an experiment with three groups of overweight kids. Each group was given a breakfast with the same number of calories. But one group ate low-fiber instant oatmeal, the second group ate high-fiber steel-cut oatmeal, and the third group ate a vegetable omelet with fruit. Each group was given a similar type of lunch and then were told to eat whenever they were hungry.

The group given the instant oatmeal ate 81 percent more food than the group that had been given the omelet, and the kids who had the steel-cut oatmeal ate 50 percent more than the omelet group. Not only did the oatmeal groups feel hungrier, but their blood tests also revealed higher levels of blood sugar, insulin, fat, and adrenaline, even though they had consumed the same amount of calories.

Dr. Ludwig's experiment focused on the effect of carbohydrates on blood sugar and appetite. Like Dr. Willett's research, it is an extremely valuable contribution to our nutritional understanding. I hope both studies make clear once and for all why simply counting calories will never lead to long-term weight loss, let alone to controlling an outsized appetite and losing your cravings for "all the wrong foods."

However, I don't want you thinking either "low-carb" or "low-fat"; rather, I want you thinking about your microbiome. Eating the kinds of carbs and fats that *support your microbiome* is the ultimate weight loss plan. Research into the microbiome was still in its infancy when Drs. Willett and Ludwig conducted their experiments. With what we know now we can see that at least part of the reason their low-carb diets succeeded was because of the ways in which these diets supported the microbiome.

THE RESEARCHERS WEIGH IN

"Our results suggest that one reason people might be eating more is because of changes in their intestinal bacteria. . . . People may be eating too much because their appetite is stronger due to low-grade inflammation they have, which could be due to changes in their gut bacteria relative to what their grandparents or someone else might have had fifty years ago."

—ANDREW GEWIRTZ, professor of microbiology and immunology, Emory University, from the journal *Science Experiments*, 2010

And so to truly understand the underlying forces driving blood sugar, insulin, appetite, and weight—to really grasp what kinds of foods affect those forces—we have to look deeper than just fats and carbs.

FAKE SURGERIES AND REAL WEIGHT LOSS

I cannot resist sharing one more crucial experiment with you, this one into the effects of gastric bypass surgery. I do not recommend gastric bypass surgery except as a last resort, and if you follow the Microbiome Diet, you are unlikely to need that last resort. But the startling results of this study make as strong a case as I could imagine for the microbiome's crucial role in weight loss.

As you may know, gastric bypass is a complex, invasive procedure in which the digestive process is surgically altered to reduce the number of calories the body is able to absorb. At least, doctors *believed* calorie reduction was the reason for the procedure's success—until researchers conducted the following groundbreaking experiment in March 2013.

Researchers compared three groups of mice. The first was given a fake surgery that had no actual effect but was performed to ensure that surgical trauma itself was not a factor. These untreated mice were then allowed unrestricted access to sweet and fatty foods, and, not surprisingly, they gained weight.

A second group of mice was given no surgery and put on a calorie-restricted diet. Not surprisingly, they lost weight.

The third group of mice was given actual gastric surgery and then allowed to eat as much as they liked. As expected, those mice also lost weight.

However, there were some significant differences between the calorie-restriction group and the gastric-bypass group. The dieting mice continued to have high insulin and high glucose levels, which, as we shall see in Chapter 2, are part of what contribute to the difficulty associated with remaining on a diet and keeping off the lost weight. When your insulin and blood sugar levels remain high, you are far more likely to crave the foods that contribute to weight gain. It's as though your whole body sets you up to fail. You might maintain your willpower for a few months or even a couple of years, but eventually your metabolism, appetite, and cravings are likely to set you up for more weight gain.

By contrast, the mice who had received the surgery had normal insulin and glucose levels. Suddenly, their bodies were setting them up not to fail but to succeed. And, indeed, after their surgeries they did not gain weight, even though they were given unlimited access to food.

So if the surgery wasn't successful simply because it restricted calories, why was it successful? The researchers speculated that the procedure had somehow "reset" the mice's hormones, perhaps by altering their microbiomes.

Now, as we shall see in Chapter 2, weight loss and metabolism are complex processes, an intricate hormonal dance that determines how blood sugar is processed, whether fat is burned or stored, and whether you feel hungry or full. When your digestive and immune system hormones go out of whack, you eat food you don't need. Then you convert that food to fat and gain weight.

By contrast, when your digestive and immune systems are in balance you eat what your body needs, burn fat, and remain at a healthy weight. And, as Robert and many of my other patients discovered, when you have achieved that vital balance you even have some leeway to indulge. That's because the crucial factor is not the number of calories you consume but rather how your body *responds* to those calories.

So yes, that bodily response is complex and multifaceted, but I can boil it down for you: *rebalance your microbiome, and the rest will follow.*

How can I assert this with such confidence? Because the research team of the gastric bypass experiment, led by Dr. Lee Kaplan, went on to test precisely that hypothesis. They transplanted the microbiota from each set of mice—fake surgery, calorie restriction, gastric bypass—to germ-free mice who had no microbiomes of their own.

Lo and behold, the germ-free mice who were colonized by the gastric-bypass microbiome lost weight, *even though they ate more* than the mice implanted with the microbiomes from the other two groups and *even though they themselves had not had the surgery.* They didn't need the surgery—they only needed a microbiome that resembled that of the mice that *did* have surgery. Apparently that was enough to alter their appetites, metabolisms, and ability to eat unrestricted amounts without gaining weight.

This sounds so unbelievable that I'm going to say it again: *even though the germ-free mice had had no surgery, no diets, and no calorie restriction, they lost weight* as soon as they were given a weight loss microbiome. Researchers concluded that the surgery had been successful not because it restricted calories but because it had somehow altered the mice's blood sugar, insulin levels—and microbiome.

The dieting mice, meanwhile, were struggling along with their calorie restriction. Their microbiomes had remained unchanged, just as their insulin and blood sugar levels had stayed the same. This is the condition that every dieter knows and hates. You starve yourself, you lose a little weight, you never stop being hungry, and the minute you start eating normally again—the minute you indulge even a little bit—the weight comes right back on.

Both as a scientist and as a physician who sees patients every day, I have known for some time that conventional approaches to diet simply do not work for most people. Even if people do lose weight following the latest diet craze, they almost never keep that weight off.

Numerous studies confirm my observation. One group of researchers found that more than 80 percent of people who lose weight regain all of it or more within the relatively short time of two years. Likewise, researchers at UCLA analyzed thirty-one long-term diet studies and discovered that about two-thirds of the dieters actually gained *more* weight in the next four or five years than they had initially lost.

Clearly, conventional approaches to diet simply do not work. But the Microbiome Diet *does* work. The more I've learned about the microbiome, the more I've come to understand it is the key to our metabolism, our weight, and our health. If you have a healthy microbiome and good intestinal health, your metabolism automatically keeps you at a healthy weight. If you have an unbalanced microbiome and poor intestinal health, you are virtually guaranteed to gain weight. Luckily for all of us, it really is that simple.

YOUR GUT HAS A MIND OF ITS OWN

The microbiome does not exist in a vacuum; it is an integral part of your gastrointestinal (GI) tract. So when we look at the connection between the microbiome and weight loss, we have to include the larger issue of overall intestinal health.

As a specialist in this field, I have always understood its importance for weight loss as well as other conditions. Over the years I have

---

THE RESEARCHERS WEIGH IN

"Bad eating habits are not sufficient to explain the worldwide explosion in obesity. . . . With each generation, there is a heavier impact on the early-life microbiome. And it means we are less and less able to metabolize the food we eat."

—MARTIN J. BLASER, chair of the Department of Medicine and a professor of microbiology, New York University School of Medicine. From the *New Yorker*, October 22, 2012 treated more than thirty thousand patients with such seemingly intractable conditions as multiple sclerosis, lupus, rheumatoid arthritis, Crohn's disease, chronic fatigue syndrome, autism, diabetes, and cancer. By helping them heal their gut and create a healthy microbiome, I was able to reduce or even eliminate their symptoms and slow or even reverse the course of the disorder, even in circumstances in which other physicians had not been able to help. Day after day I saw evidence in my practice of the wisdom of Hippocrates, founder of Western medicine, who taught us that "All disease begins in the gut." I say, all health begins in the gut as well.

Over the past few years an explosion of scientific and popular articles confirms my belief as our understanding of the digestive system continues to evolve. When I was in medical school they called the gut "the blind tube." Now we understand that it's just the opposite: Your gut has a mind of its own. A pioneering book on gut health published in 1998 by Michael Gershon, MD, was actually entitled *The Second Brain*.

The more we learn about the gut, the more its special intelligence becomes clear. Did you know, for example, there are more nerves in the gut than in the spinal column? These nerves transmit important messages to and from the brain, and a growing body of research suggests we cannot fully treat mental and psychiatric problems without taking the gut into account.

That's because the relationship between the brain and the gut is very much a two-way street. When you are feeling stressed, anxious, or angry, your brain triggers a response from your adrenal system to flood your body with stress chemicals. These chemicals disrupt your digestion, often producing such symptoms as gas, bloating, heartburn (gastroesophageal reflux disease, or GERD), and, in the long run, weight gain. (We'll learn more about this gut-brain relationship in Chapter 7, "Stress Can Make You Fat.")

Your gut produces neurotransmitters, the brain chemicals you need to feel calm, balanced, optimistic, energized, and focused. But when your GI tract is not functioning properly it cannot synthesize enough of these crucial chemicals.

For example, *serotonin* is a crucial neurotransmitter for feeling optimistic and self-confident as well as a critical component of our ability to get good sleep. When your serotonin levels are disrupted you might feel hopeless, unsure of your own abilities, and blue while also struggling with anxiety, agitation, and insomnia. In more serious cases low serotonin levels can lead to a diagnosis of depression.

Yet some 95 percent of our body's serotonin is located in the gut, where it helps regulate digestion. If our GI tract isn't functioning properly, it can't produce the serotonin we need either for good digestion *or* for feeling good.

Your gut is also a crucial part of your immune system: Some 70 to 80 percent of the immune system is found within the gut. This makes sense when you consider that one of your immune system's main functions is to protect you from bacteria, viruses, or toxins that might lurk in your food. So when your GI tract is not in good condition you are more prone to colds, infections, acne, and a host of other minor problems, not to mention more serious illnesses.

In other words, your intestinal health is absolutely crucial to your metabolism, your appetite, your cravings, and your weight, not to mention your mood, appearance, energy levels, and ability to withstand stress and infection.

THE BENEFITS OF "MICROBIOME MEDICINE" AND GUT HEALING

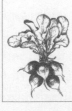

- Fast, dramatic, permanent weight loss
- Vastly improved mental focus, emotional state, and energy levels
- Improved response to stress
- Healthier immune system
- Beautiful, glowing skin
- Restored hair growth
- Renewed sense of vibrancy and vitality

THE ULTIMATE SOCIAL NETWORK

The exciting thing about the microbiome is the way it represents a genuine paradigm shift—in weight loss, in our understanding of health and disease, and in our sense of our own identities.

We have already seen how rapidly the microbiome is transforming our view of weight loss. First we had calorie counting, then we had low-fat diets, then low-carb diets, and, most recently, we had diets based on combating inflammation, often by withdrawing certain inflammatory foods from our diets. Some of these approaches had merit, whereas some were completely off base. But none of them got to the root of the problem: the health and function of our microbiome, supported by a healthy, high-functioning digestive system. Fix the microbiome and repair the gut—as the Microbiome Diet helps you to do—and, almost effortlessly, weight loss will follow.

The paradigm shift is no less important in medicine. When I was in medical school we were taught to divide the human anatomy into discrete systems: the immune system, the digestive system, the nervous system. It's not unusual for a patient who complains of depression to be referred to a psychiatrist or psychologist, whereas the same patient, experiencing bloating, gas, constipation, and weight gain, would be referred to an internist, a nutritionist, or perhaps a gastroenterologist. In conventional medicine it is a rare doctor who will view the depression and digestive symptoms as potentially stemming from the same cause.

Yet once you understand the powerful role of the microbiome you begin to see that the human body really is a single system with a tremendous amount of "cross-talk" among all the different aspects of our body. As we will see in Chapter 2, an imbalanced microbiome might be at least partly responsible for the depression by disrupting your intestinal production of serotonin, a chemical that enables you to feel hopeful, confident, and calm. At the same time, that same imbalanced microbiome is disrupting your digestive, immune, and endocrine systems and ultimately cuing your body to store fat. Both the depression and the weight gain might well stem from the same cause.

As we will also see in Chapter 2, your immune system is involved in this interaction as well, creating inflammation that attacks both your gut and your brain, worsening both your depression and your weight gain. An imbalanced microbiome thus leads to multiple symptoms, such as weight gain, digestive problems, immune issues, low energy, foggy concentration, anxiety, and depression.

The Microbiome Diet allows you to address all of these systems at the same time simply by supporting your microbiome and, in the process, healing your gut. I know this approach will do for you what it has done for Robert and hundreds of my other patients: it will help you take the pounds off and ensure that you can *keep* them off while ultimately maintaining only 70 percent compliance. But I want to encourage you to see your weight loss, like Robert's, as an aspect of overall healing that will transform many aspects of your health.

The important role of the microbiome is slowly but surely being recognized by the world of medicine. In January 2014 the *Proceedings* of the prestigious Mayo Clinic published a primer on how physicians might incorporate scientific research on the microbiome into their clinical practice. The article expressed my own feelings about the crucial implications of the microbiome for human health, saying that "in a short time, understanding the basic concepts about the interactions between humans and their microbiome will be as important to clinicians as understanding concepts of genetics or germ theory."

The most important paradigm shift, however, is in our view of what it means to be human. Contrary to what most of us have grown up believing, we are not autonomous, independent, self-regulated beings, free of dependence from any outside systems or organisms. Instead, we are interdependent ecologies responsible, like Horton, for safeguarding the extraordinary world that lives within us. The microbiome is the ultimate social network, a community in continual communication with itself and with us. Although we are used to thinking of bacteria and microbes as negative, as the source of disease and infection, our new understanding shows us that microbial life can also be a source of health, well-being, and weight loss.

In Chapter 2 I explain exactly how a healthy microbiome supports weight loss, whereas an imbalanced microbiome leads to weight gain. Then, in Part II of this book, I share with you my own adaptation of the "Four Rs"—the protocol that practitioners of functional medicine use to restore intestinal health. As you will see, the first three weeks of the Microbiome Diet focus on healing foods and supplements that will put both your microbiome and your entire digestive system on the path to optimal health.

In Part III, I prepare you for the next phase of the Microbiome Diet, which gives you a metabolic boost even while allowing you to widen your diet somewhat and to maintain only 90 percent compliance. You learn how stress can make you fat while discovering that focused eating—mindful, appreciative, and full of pleasure—can aid your weight loss efforts.

In Part IV, I set you up for a lifetime of a healthy gut and healthy microbiome, enabling you to maintain only 70 percent compliance. At long last you will able to eat indulgently while staying at a healthy weight as long as you continue to support your microbiome.

Finally, in Part V, I give you all the tools you need to follow the Microbiome Diet. I explain the Microbiome Superfoods, Superspices, and Supersupplements—the foods, spices, and supplements that will support your microbiome, heal your intestinal tract, rev up your metabolism, and help you achieve both a healthy weight and better overall health. I tell you exactly how to stock your kitchen, and I provide you with weekly shopping lists. I share with you meal plans and recipes to carry you through Phase 1 and Phase 2 of the diet. I even give you weekly work plans, helping you prepare foods ahead of time and showing you how to refrigerate or freeze leftovers so as to cut down on cooking time throughout the week. Last but not least, I explain how to approach Phase 3, during which you create your own meal plans and enjoy only 70 percent compliance, with the freedom to indulge in other types of food up to 30 percent of the time.

This is an exciting journey, and I'm eager to help you get started. Let me leave you with these inspiring words from researcher Sarkis K. Mazmanian of the California Institute of Technology, as quoted in an article in *Scientific American*. Mazmanian explains why it has taken us so long to grasp the central role of the microbiome, the "forgotten organ" of the human anatomy:

> Our narcissism held us back. We tended to think we had all the functions required for our health. But just because microbes are foreign, just because we acquired them throughout life, doesn't mean they're any less a fundamental part of us.

two

YOUR FAT IS NOT YOUR FAULT

HAVE YOU EVER FELT AS THOUGH YOUR METABOLISM HAS BEEN HIJACKED, that your body is simply not under your control?

Have you ever felt as though you could just look at food and gain weight and then wondered why your friend could eat as much as she wants and stay slim?

Have you ever felt as though you were the prisoner of your own cravings and hungers, that something other than you was driving you to eat foods you knew were bad for you but you simply couldn't resist? Or that you are hungry almost all the time, even after you have just eaten?

Have you ever felt as though all your weight loss efforts were being secretly sabotaged from within?

These feelings are not excuses, rationalizations, or signs of poor willpower. They represent your body's awareness that *you are not just a person—you are an ecosystem.* You contain within you an entire microscopic world whose biology is central to *your* biology. Although, like Horton's neighbors, you may be unaware of these tiny organisms living within your body, they affect you nonetheless. The state of your microbiome determines:

- **What kinds of foods you crave**—sweets and starches or healthy fruits and vegetables
- **When you feel hungry**—all the time or only when you really need more nourishment
- **How your food is metabolized**—as stored-up fat that collects around your waist and abdomen or as energy that is used for your day's needs so that even if you eat somewhat indulgently, you never gain weight.

So in this chapter I'm going to show you exactly how and why improving the health of your microbiome is the single-best thing you can do for your appetite, metabolism, and your weight.

I honestly think you will enjoy following the Microbiome Diet. The recipes are amazing, devised by a wellness chef, and the food combinations are designed to leave you feeling full and satisfied. But,

---

THE MICROBIOME: KEY WEIGHT LOSS FACTS

- Supporting your microbiome frees you of hunger, cravings, and the feeling that your metabolism has simply "gone out of control."
- You can change your microbiome incredibly quickly. Within just a few hours you can shift into an unhealthy state that creates weight gain. Within just a few weeks you can restore it to a healthy state.
- Supporting your microbiome also affects your brain. A healthy microbiome can go a long way toward ending depression, anxiety, brain fog, fatigue, and the inability to concentrate.
- A healthy microbiome can clear your skin, improve your hair, and boost your energy levels.

- Once your microbiome is balanced you can "eat like a thin person," occasionally indulging in desserts and rich foods, because your metabolism is so healthy.

as with all my patients, I believe if you understand what we're doing here, you'll feel a lot more excited and motivated about undertaking this weight loss journey with me. So let's take a look at some of the extraordinary research linking the microbiome with weight loss as you get to know your microbiome a little better.

"WHY AM I ALWAYS HUNGRY?"

My patient Kendall was always hungry.

"I don't know what it is," she told me, almost in tears. "I used to eat oatmeal with sliced bananas for breakfast, because I read that the oatmeal was good for my cholesterol and the bananas were full of potassium. Then I read that low-carb was the best way to lose weight, so I switched to eggs, whole-grain toast, juice, and tea. I always have a healthy lunch—a big salad with grilled chicken and lots of vegetables. And I stick to a healthy dinner—broiled fish and a sweet potato and steamed broccoli or kale or something like that. I *know* that should be enough—I know it! But I can't lose weight, and I feel like I'm starving all the time!"

Kendall told me that sometimes she had the willpower to stick to her regime, but often she didn't. She found herself craving macaroni and cheese, a piece of toasted pound cake, or a bowl of chocolate ice cream. Whether she resisted these temptations or not she felt as though nothing ever really satisfied her.

Kendall had gained fifteen pounds in the past year, "and I was already about fifteen pounds too heavy before that," she told me. "I know I should be eating better, but honestly, Doctor Kellman, I don't even see why I should, because once I stuck to my low-carb diet for three whole months, and all I lost was three pounds. I can only lose one pound a month? What in the world is *wrong* with me?"

As I questioned Kendall more closely I could see there were many signs pointing to an imbalanced microbiome and impaired intestinal health. But when I broached this possibility to her, she shook her head.

"I can tell you that nothing is wrong with my digestion," she said emphatically. "I never have gas or bloating or anything like that, and

I never have indigestion. My bowel movements are very regular—I go once or twice a day, very easily. Whatever else is wrong with me, it isn't that."

I got the questionnaire I ask all patients to fill out and showed Kendall the symptoms she had checked off: headache, difficulty concentrating, occasional eczema, mild anxiety, some trouble sleeping. Her eyes widened in surprise.

"Do you mean to tell me that those things are because of my *digestion*?" she asked skeptically.

"Sometimes digestive issues show up where you don't expect them," I explained. "After all, you are one body—one whole, made up of many interconnected systems that are always in communication. And your microbiome is an incredible social network that gets into the conversation as well. The combination of your weight gain, your appetite, and the symptoms you mentioned tells me both your microbiome and your gut are out of balance and need some support."

Kendall was even more surprised when I told her that some elements in her "healthy" diet were not so healthy after all, at least not while her microbiome and intestinal system were in distress. Because she had been failing to nourish her microbiome, her microbiome had become imbalanced. This imbalanced microbiome had created three problems.

First, an imbalanced microbiome had created all sorts of disregulation in Kendall's immune system. As a result, she was experiencing *inflammation*, a type of immune system response that can lead to weight gain.

Second, her imbalanced microbiome had created a problem known as *intestinal permeability*, or, to use its more popular name, *leaky gut*. Leaky gut also causes your immune system to react badly to foods that would otherwise be healthy. This produces even more inflammation and, thus, further contributes to weight gain.

Finally, Kendall's imbalanced microbiome was also disrupting her hormonal balance. As a result the hormones that made Kendall feel hungry or full were seriously out of whack. This made it hard for Kendall to stop eating when she had actually consumed enough food, so once again her body was cuing her to gain weight.

Besides causing Kendall to gain weight, inflammation was also creating her symptoms: the headaches, difficulty concentrating, skin problems, anxiety, and sleep problems. So in order to stop the inflammation, heal the symptoms, and reverse the weight gain, we had to rebalance Kendall's microbiome.

At the same time we had to figure out which foods she was temporarily overreacting to—foods that were also setting off an immune response. I knew that eggs are often a reactive food that can set off an immune response. So is gluten, a protein found in wheat, rye, barley, and many other grains and often added to many foods, including ketchup, canned soups, and protein bars. Kendall's eggs and toast were, therefore, likely to be causing her problems along with the milk she put into her tea (dairy is often a reactive food) and the soy sauce on her broiled fish (soy is also reactive for many people, and most soy sauce contains gluten).

So, I told Kendall, there were a lot of things going wrong: food sensitivities, leaky gut, hormonal imbalances, immune disregulation, and inflammation. But the ultimate cause of all these problems was an imbalanced microbiome, which was sabotaging her metabolism and ultimately causing both her symptoms and her weight gain.

I'll explain all of these factors in more detail throughout this chapter. But I'll share the solution right now. Kendall went on the Microbiome Diet, which in Phase 1 kept her away from reactive foods for three weeks while focusing on healing foods to rebalance her microbiome and restore her intestinal health. In Phase 2, when her system was stronger and more balanced, she was able to add in some more foods and maintain only 90 percent compliance. And after four weeks of Phase 2 Kendall could move on to Phase 3, the lifetime maintenance phase, which provided her with plenty of healing foods and supplements to support her microbiome and her digestion while still allowing her to maintain only 70 percent compliance.

Over the course of a year Kendall let go of most of her unwanted weight, and she is optimistic about losing the rest. But even before she had lost her first ten pounds Kendall felt like a changed woman.

"I'm not hungry anymore, except when it really is time to eat," she told me triumphantly. "I don't think about food hardly at all. Sure, I love a good meal, but it's not the highlight of my day anymore. It's not the thing I'm always focused on. I feel like before I was a prisoner, and now I've been let out of jail."

HUNGRY NO MORE!

There are so many ways that your microbiome affects your hunger that I am only going to focus on a few. But I want you to understand at least something about this complex relationship so you will see why I say supporting your microbiome will help regulate your appetite and free you from feeling, like Kendall, "always hungry."

One of the most fascinating microbes in the human microbiome is *helicobacter pylori*, or *h. pylori*. Over the past several years *h. pylori* has gotten lots of bad press because it is one of the primary causes of peptic ulcers. As a result scientists and physicians engaged in a largely successful campaign to rid the human body of *h. pylori* without stopping to consider whether there might also be some collateral damage.

It turns out that *h. pylori* regulates acid production in the stomach — a useful task, as we need stomach acid to digest our food as well as to neutralize viruses and other toxic invaders that might enter our bodies through our mouths. Even more significant for dieters, however, *h. pylori* also helps to regulate *ghrelin*, the hormone that tells your brain when your body needs to eat.

A person whose microbiome includes *h. pylori* can expect a decrease in ghrelin after eating. As a result, hunger dissipates until it is time for the next meal. For obvious reasons, that is how your body is supposed to work.

H. pylori also helps you regulate the levels of another hormone, *leptin*. With a healthy microbiome, leptin rises as ghrelin falls, signaling fullness, suppressing your appetite, and giving you a boost of energy.

SYMPTOMS OF AN IMBALANCED MICROBIOME

abdominal pain	hair loss and dull, lifeless hair
aging too rapidly	headache
anal itching	infections
allergies	joint pain
anxiety	lightheadedness
arthritis	low energy
bloating and gas	memory problems
brain fog	muscle pain
constipation	nausea
depressed mood	poor skin color
diarrhea	rashes and other skin reactions
difficulty focusing	sexual dysfunction or lowered
dry skin	sex drive
eczema	swelling of ankles
fatigue	tingling/numbing in hands and feet
feeling too full, that food is just sitting in your stomach and not being digested	

But if you don't have *h. pylori* in your microbiome—and at this point many of us don't—your microbiome has more difficulty shutting off that hunger signal and turning on the fullness signal. A recent study of ninety-two veterans showed that those who had been treated with antibiotics to eliminate *h. pylori* gained more weight than their peers who had not been treated.

Because of the increased use of antibiotics, more and more children are growing up without *h. pylori* in their microbiomes. Some researchers speculate that this might be the reason behind the childhood obesity epidemic. NYU researcher Martin J. Blaser, by having a team from his laboratory administer antibiotics to mice in dosages comparable to those received by children with ear infections, demonstrated that antibiotics lead to weight gain. Even though the mice ate exactly the same food as before, their weight suddenly skyrocketed. The disruption to their microbiomes caused them to experience every dieter's nightmare: absorbing more calories from the same amount of food.

We shouldn't be surprised. Until recently some three-fourths of all antibiotics given in the United States were fed not to people but to cows, pigs, and poultry—not to treat them for diseases but to fatten them up. The livestock and poultry industries didn't know *why* antibiotics worked so well, but they did know the meds made their animals fatter. Clearly they make us fatter too, by increasing both our body fat percentage as well as the livestock we eat.

By the time the average American kid turns eighteen he or she has been given between ten and twenty courses of antibiotics. In the developed world—where the obesity epidemic has already kicked off—children are given antibiotics an average of every other year. Altering our microbiomes seems to be fattening us as efficiently as if we were so many cows. The good news is that supporting your microbiome can reverse that effect and allow you to take the weight off.

HOW THE MICROBIOME AFFECTS YOUR WEIGHT

Because your body is a complex organism with lots of interaction and "cross-talk" between systems, disentangling the many ways in which the microbiome affects your weight can be challenging. The following chart is by no means comprehensive, but it does give you a quick summary.

Let's take a closer look.

INFLAMMATION AND YOUR MICROBIOME

Inflammation is a reaction from your immune system that creates all sorts of health problems throughout your body. When your immune system attacks a genuine invader—say, the bacteria that causes pneumonia or a toxin that might poison you to death—inflammation flares up as a kind of collateral damage, as though the defense force that had been mobilized to neutralize the enemy shot up a few neighboring buildings as well.

IMBALANCED MICROBIOME	BALANCED MICROBIOME
Weight Gain, Obesity	**Weight Loss, Healthy Weight**
• Provokes inflammation • Creates insulin resistance • Worsens food sensitivities and leaky gut • Creates hunger • Cues your genes to hold onto fat	• Regulates the harvest of calories and "energy extraction" from your food • Produces "short-chain fatty acids," which have incredible weight loss properties • Decreases inflammation • Tells your genes to burn fat rather than store it

When there really is a toxic invader—an acute, temporary, fixable problem—a healthy immune system will zap it. With the danger gone, the inflammation subsides.

But when your body is continually subjected to stress or danger, even a low-grade stress or a mild danger, it can go into a chronic state of inflammation. Because danger never really goes away, the inflammation never goes away either. And the longer inflammation sticks around, the worse your health becomes.

In fact, chronic inflammation is one of the gravest health problems that we face in this country. At worst it can lead to autoimmune conditions (including rheumatoid arthritis, multiple sclerosis, lupus), diabetes, heart disease, and cancer. Even mild inflammatory symptoms can be painful (see the list on page 37), particularly because they include persistent, stubborn weight gain. If you've tried and failed to lose weight, chances are inflammation is fighting you every step of the way, cuing your body to hold onto fat no matter how little you eat or how much you exercise.

Many factors can cause inflammation, including stress (too many obligations, not enough downtime); medications (both over-the-counter and prescription); and a diet high in sweets, starches, and unhealthy fats. Dr. Paresh Dandona, a professor at the State University of New York at Buffalo and the head of the Diabetes-Endocrinology Center of West New York, has confirmed in a particularly dramatic way the inflammatory role of diet.

In 2004 Dr. Dandona measured the effects of a typical fast food breakfast. He asked his research subjects to consume two breakfast sandwiches—one egg, ham, and cheese, the other sausage on a muffin—along with two hash brown patties. Then he measured their blood levels of c-reactive protein (CRP), a marker for inflammation. To Dandona's surprise, his subjects' rate of inflammation skyrocketed within minutes—and remained high for hours.

Dr. Dandona had expected *some* reaction from the inflammatory food, but no one had ever documented such a rapid response. Eventually Dandona discovered that foods high in processed sugar, refined carbs, and unhealthy fats encourage the growth of certain types of gut bacteria. Because the life span of a microbe is only twenty minutes, the "bad" bacteria begin to overwhelm the "good" bacteria as soon as they get a taste of that unhealthy fat and starch. The bad bacteria quickly produce a substance called *endotoxin*, which provokes the immune system into a defensive reaction—that is, inflammation.

Here is where your metabolism comes in. The inflammation triggers an overproduction of insulin, which cues your body to stop burning fat and start storing it. Inflammation also imbalances your leptin signals, which, as we have seen, makes it harder for you to feel full.

Now, if you're trying to lose weight, this metabolic change seems like the ultimate insult. *Why is my body working against me?* you might ask. *Why is it holding onto fat? Why won't it let me feel full?*

To answer those questions I'd like you to imagine that you are one of the earliest humans on earth. Perhaps you're huddled by the fire during a cold, endless winter. Perhaps you're walking through the woods on a blazing hot day, desperately foraging for food. Perhaps you're trekking across the tundra with your fellow villagers, a baby strapped to your back, a child at your side, hoping that you and your loved ones survive the long, uncertain journey.

Although you are not facing any immediate danger, like a bandit or a saber-tooth tiger—no need for fight or flight!—you *are* in a chronic state of low-grade stress. As a result you suffer from chronic, low-grade inflammation. And that inflammation cues your immune system to alter your metabolism.

Remember, your body is in crisis. By altering your metabolism, your body is trying to help you survive in the best way it knows how: holding onto every last ounce of weight and particularly every last ounce of body fat. After all, food is scarce, you need your body fat to keep warm, and you don't always know where your next meal is coming from. If you do encounter a food source, you don't want to eat a few bites, fill up, and burn your body fat to maintain your slim figure; instead, you want to gorge yourself until you're stuffed, flood your blood with insulin to process all those extra calories, convert those calories into fat, and hold onto that fat for dear life.

Of course, if you are reading this book, you are probably *not* facing a chronic threat of starvation. More likely, you are desperate to let go of the extra pounds and excess body fat that are threatening your health and well-being, and you would love to naturally stop eating when you no longer need the extra food. But the connection is clear: A body under stress sends messages to hold onto every extra ounce of fat. Whether your stress is caused by a trek across the tundra, too many deadlines, or an ongoing family problem, your body is getting the same message and responding in the same way: by holding onto fat.

Luckily, there is a solution: Heal the inflammation, restore your microbiome to a healthier ecology, and reset your metabolism to burn fat rather than store it. Your first step is to stop eating the kinds of sweets, starches, and unhealthy fats that feed those disruptive microbes. Switch to the kinds of foods that will support a healthier type of bacteria—the Microbiome Superfoods that are high in fiber and healthy fats—and you've just taken a huge step toward success.

YOUR MICROBIOME AND INSULIN RESISTANCE

Groundbreaking research conducted by Patrice Cani at the Catholic University of Louvain in Brussels, Belgium, shows us exactly why we need a diet that supports our microbiome. To mimic the effects of an unhealthy diet, Cani dosed his mice with endotoxins. As expected, the mice gained weight.

They also developed *insulin resistance*, a condition in which cells fail to respond to normal amounts of insulin. Cells require insulin to absorb glucose (made from carbs), fatty acids (made from fats), and amino acids (made from protein). So without enough insulin your cells would starve. In fact, this is what happens to diabetics. No matter how much they eat, if they couldn't supplement the missing insulin, they would literally starve to death.

When cells become resistant to insulin, however, they require ever-increasing amounts of it to absorb glucose. As the process breaks down, more and more sugar is left to circulate in the bloodstream rather than being absorbed by the cells that need it. You feel the desire to eat partly to compensate for all that nourishment your body is not getting. Your pancreas works harder and harder to make the extra insulin, putting you at risk for diabetes. And instead of being converted into energy for your cells, the excess sugar and fats in your bloodstream are stored as fat, either in the body or in the liver. Fatty liver used to be seen only among alcoholics, but now, as part of the obesity epidemic, we are seeing "nonalcoholic fatty liver" among obese adults and children as well.

As we might expect, Cani's obese, insulin-resistant mice did develop diabetes. And when he gave his mice unhealthy fats instead of endotoxins, he triggered the same process:

unhealthy fats ➡ endotoxins ➡ inflammation ➡ insulin resistance ➡ obesity/risk of diabetes

Now here's the good news. As soon as Cani gave the mice *oligosaccharides*—soluble plant fibers found in onions, leeks, garlic, asparagus, jicama, and Jerusalem artichokes—the whole cascade was averted. No endotoxins. No inflammation. No insulin resistance. And no weight gain.

Why? Because the beneficial bacteria in the microbiome flourish when given oligosaccharides, which are a type of prebiotic. As we have seen, prebiotics nourish the healthy bacteria in our microbiome, and indeed, when Cani's mice were given prebiotics, their healthy bacteria began to outnumber the disruptive bacteria. It was as though the well-fed healthy bacteria were now able to force the bad bacteria to leave the neighborhood. Consuming prebiotics means microbial balance is restored. Inflammation subsides. Good health and healthy weight are the result.

And yes, the Microbiome Diet is full of delicious oligosaccharides as well as other types of prebiotics that help you maintain a healthy microbial balance. Like Cani's mice, you can avert metabolic danger by starving the bad bacteria while feeding the good bacteria. It is literally a recipe for weight loss.

By the way, Dr. Dandona got the same result with his human subjects when he added fresh orange juice to their inflammatory breakfasts. The good bacteria fed on the orange juice, gaining the strength to drive away the bad bacteria and their endotoxins. I think there are far better prebiotics than orange juice, which raises other nutritional concerns, so there's no OJ on the Microbiome Diet. But I am always happy to read studies that affirm the power of the microbiome!

FOOD SENSITIVITIES, LEAKY GUT, AND WEIGHT GAIN

There is one more way that microbiome-induced inflammation can disrupt your metabolism and promote weight gain: *intestinal permeability*, a.k.a. leaky gut.

Let's look for a moment at a gut that is *not* leaky—a healthy, impermeable intestine. That intestine receives partially digested food from your stomach, drawing the nutrients from that food in microscopic amounts. The nutrients pass through the lining of your intestinal wall, known as the *epithelium*. Eventually they are released into the bloodstream, which transports that life-giving nourishment throughout the body.

For this process to work correctly the intestinal walls need what are known as *tight junctions*. The epithelial cells must fit together snugly so only microscopic amounts of nourishment pass through.

When these tight junctions come apart, however, the intestine becomes permeable, creating leaky gut. Partially digested food can seep through the epithelium, where it is not supposed to go. When the immune system detects these intruders, it doesn't realize they are only partially digested foods; it considers them toxic invaders and mobilizes for the attack.

Your immune system also develops *antibodies* so it can recognize each intruder the next time. It's as though your body were making a list of potential dangers: dairy products, soy, gluten, eggs. . . .

So now we have two problems: your immune system reacts negatively to a food that might otherwise be healthy, and your leaky intestine isn't operating up to par. If you eat a reactive food often enough, your immune system ends up on permanent alert, and chronic, low-grade inflammation is the result. Insulin resistance follows, along with a fat-storing metabolism, excess body fat, weight gain, and the threat of diabetes.

To make matters worse, inflammation itself can create leaky gut. And abdominal fat is inflammatory, as is all that extra insulin you are pumping through your system. Talk about a vicious cycle!

Here's another vicious cycle: the antibodies your immune system creates are programmed to seek out a specific invader—for example, dairy. If your immune system creates too many "antidairy" antibodies, you will actually begin to crave dairy *because your antibodies are seeking it*. They want to destroy the food and you want to eat it, but both you and your antibodies are fixated on a food that, because of your immune system reaction, will cause you to gain weight, develop symptoms, and suffer more inflammation.

This is why so many of my patients feel like prisoners of their cravings and their appetites. Their entire biology is set up to want the wrong foods. The disruptive parts of their microbiome crave unhealthy fats, sweets, and starches. Their immune systems create antibodies that crave certain foods, and then they overreact to those very foods. Their leptin signals are turned down so they can never feel full, while their ghrelin signals are turned up so they must always feel hungry. If they happen to also have yeast overgrowth—a common result of an imbalanced microbiome—then the yeast in their bodies also craves sugar.

Luckily you can turn this process around and free yourself from your cravings. Pulling certain foods from your diet, at least temporarily, helps reduce the inflammation and get rid of the antibodies, while repairing your gut wall gets your whole system back on track.

And guess what? Besides all its other functions, your microbiome provides crucial support for a strong gut wall. In fact, research has shown that without a healthy microbiome the epithelium will not function. It will remain semidormant, and, because 70 percent of our immune system is in the epithelium, our immune system will not function properly either. Once again a healthy microbiome is the key.

THE ENERGY HARVEST

Your microbiome doesn't just cue your immune system; it also cues your digestive system, helping to determine how many calories you harvest from the food and beverages you consume. Some bacteria extract more energy out of food than do others. That's part of the reason why one person gains weight with every extra bite while her best friend can have three desserts a week and not put on a pound. Balancing your microbiome will help you get the right amount of calories from the foods you consume and will ultimately enable you to maintain only 70 percent compliance while still remaining at a healthy weight.

SHORT-CHAIN FATTY ACIDS: CREATING A METABOLIC BOOST

Short-chain fatty acids (SCFAs) don't have an especially glamorous name, but they are one of your microbiome's most potent weapons for fighting fat, preserving health, and revving up your metabolism.

SCFAs are produced when the bacteria in your microbiome feed on oligosaccharides, the fibers in various vegetables that make it all the way to your colon "undigested." When you eat onions, leeks, asparagus, jicama, or Jerusalem artichokes (our Microbiome Superfoods), it's as though you're sending dinner down to your microbiome, whose bacteria feast on these fibers by fermenting them. The by-products of that fermentation, the SCFAs, include acetate (acetic acid) and butyrate (butyric acid) as well as B vitamins and vitamin K. One of your dietary goals is to eat enough oligosaccharides and other prebiotics to keep the good bacteria in your microbiome well fed and happy.

Butyrate is a kind of metabolic wonder drug. It improves insulin sensitivity while increasing energy expenditure—the amount of your fat that is burned off as energy. It modulates your immune system to protect you against infection and disease while supporting the integrity of your epithelium, thus preventing leaky gut. High levels of butyrate also offer effective prevention against inflammation.

Acetate reduces inflammation too. And both compounds increase mitochondrial function. The mitochondrion is the part of the cell where energy is produced and fat is burned. Inflammation can

---

Cutting-Edge Studies:
The Microbiome and Weight Loss

A wide variety of research has shown that prebiotics support the microbiome and, therefore, produce a metabolic boost:

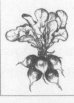

- Feeding mice a probiotic apparently *blocked* weight gain. The probiotic also helped decrease inflammation and improve the tight junctions in the epithelial walls.
- Other studies have revealed that short-chain fatty acids block inflammation in a variety of ways while also protecting the epithelial walls.
- Vitamin B, a by-product of the microbiota that ferment plant fibers, seems to decrease intestinal permeability.
- Acetate acid significantly improves epithelial function and decreases insulin resistance while helping subjects lose weight, decrease cholesterol, and lower their triglycerides.

easily damage vulnerable mitochondria, which can lead ultimately to fat storage.

So short-chain fatty acids help your metabolism by affecting the mitochondria in two ways. First, they turn on the fat-burning activity of the mitochondria. Second, they help the mitochondria recover from inflammation so they can then burn more fat. If you want a metabolic boost, improve your microbiome so it can produce more of these "weight loss wonder drugs"!

TRANSFORM YOUR MICROBIOME . . . AND YOUR METABOLISM

In September 2013 a very exciting study was published in *Science* magazine demonstrating the extraordinary power of the microbiome to transform your metabolism. I'd like to talk you through the study because it provides dramatic evidence of how an unhealthy microbiome almost guarantees weight gain, while a healthy microbiome sets you up for an ideal, healthy weight. For those of you who have felt frustrated by how quickly you seem to gain weight or how you cannot stray from a rigid diet even a little bit, this study clarifies that once your microbiome is healthy, your metabolism will work for you, not against you.

Vanessa K. Ridaura, a graduate student at Washington University School of Medicine in St. Louis, conducted this study. Ridaura wanted to explore the extent of the microbiome's influence on a person's tendency to gain or lose weight. To make sure that genetics were not an issue, she began with four pairs of female twins, each of whom by definition shared the same genes. However, in each pair one twin was lean while the other was obese. Same genes, different microbiomes—different weight.

Ridaura then transplanted some of the fecal matter (because it contains intestinal bacteria) from the humans to some germ-free mice that had no microbiomes of their own. The mice that got transplants from the obese twins became obese. The mice that got transplants from the lean twins remained lean.

If Ridaura had stopped there, she would already have gone a long way toward demonstrating that a healthy microbiome can help preserve a healthy weight, while an imbalanced microbiome has a powerful tendency to produce obesity. But Ridaura went even further. She housed mice from both groups—those that had gotten the "lean" transplants and those that had gotten the "obese" ones—in the same area. When they were living with the "lean" mice, the mice that had gotten "obese" transplants *did not become obese*.

Why not? Because, as Ridaura's experiment confirmed and as other experiments have demonstrated, we share our microbiomes with the people whom we encounter, and we share even more of our microbiomes with the people we are closest to. People who live together exchange bacteria all the time. For example, in a study of two roller derby teams, the members of each team shared some similarities in their microbiomes.

In Ridaura's experiment a specific microbe known as bacteroides SPP passed from the mice that had gotten the "lean" transplant to the mice that had gotten the "obese" transplant. The bacteroides SPP seemed to actually protect the "obese transplant" mice against obesity.

What's fascinating is that the colonization did not work in the opposite direction. The mice that had gotten the "obese" transplants did not transmit their "fat-producing" bacteria to the thin mice.

This is such hopeful news! Even though an imbalanced microbiome creates such disastrous consequences for our weight and health, it is relatively easy for us to overpower the bad bacteria and support the good bacteria. The bad guys lose, the good guys win, and obesity is defeated.

But here's the catch: Ridaura's experiment depended upon feeding her mice the correct diet. To resist the dangers of the "obese" microbiome—the one that, all things being equal, would create obesity after a transplant—the mice had to be eating a high-fiber diet that was relatively low in unhealthy fats.

This makes complete sense when we remember Dandona's and Cani's studies. The wrong type of bacteria feed on unhealthy fats—

that's why Dandona's subjects showed a skyrocketing incidence of inflammation soon after they ate the greasy breakfast food. The right type of bacteria feed on fiber, a powerful prebiotic. That's why both Dandona's humans and Cani's mice could resist the inflammatory endotoxins if they were given foods that nourished the good bacteria—orange juice in Dandona's case, oligosaccharides in Cani's.

In other words, by feeding the mice their own version of the Microbiome Diet, Ridaura ensured they could resist the dangers of bad bacteria by nourishing their own good bacteria.

This is why I don't want you counting calories on the Microbiome Diet and why you will be able to maintain only 70 percent compliance once your microbiome is in good shape. As long as you are eating the Microbiome Superfoods that support your microbiome and are not eating too many foods that are bad for it, you can eat comfortably and even somewhat indulgently while still remaining thin. When you run into problems—whatever your calorie count—is when you feed the bad bacteria and starve the good ones. That's why even people on a relatively healthy diet sometimes struggle with losing weight; as healthy as their diets might be, they are not doing enough to nourish their good bacteria. And it's why some people seem to have room for a certain amount of indulgence even while remaining trim. Because they *are* nourishing their good bacteria, they are also effectively preventing inflammation, thereby avoiding the whole set of vicious cycles we explored earlier in this chapter.

THE DIET THAT WILL CHANGE YOUR LIFE

I think of the Microbiome Diet as the royal road to health. Besides helping you lose weight, it has extraordinary healing powers for all sorts of conditions. When you balance your microbiome your skin will glow, your hair will become healthier, and you'll have boatloads of energy. Your mood will improve—a healthy microbiome combats anxiety and depression. Your brain will feel focused and laser-sharp: a healthy microbiome clears away brain fog.

THE MICROBIOME DIET AT A GLANCE

PHASE 1: THE FOUR Rs

Heal Your Gut for Healthy Weight Loss

This phase of the Microbiome Diet is based on the protocol that physicians use to restore their patients to intestinal health, which we call the Four Rs:

THE FOUR Rs

▶ **Remove** the unhealthy bacteria and the foods that unbalance the microbiome.

▶ **Replace** the digestive enzymes that you need for optimal digestion.

▶ **Reinoculate** with *probiotics* (intestinal bacteria) and *prebiotics* (foods and supplements that nourish this bacteria and keep it healthy).

▶ **Repair** the lining of your intestinal walls, which have likely become permeable and are releasing partially digested food into your bloodstream—with disastrous results.

In this phase of the Microbiome Diet, you will avoid sugar, eggs, soy, gluten, and dairy. You will avoid artificial colors and preservatives while loading up on healing foods that contain *inulin, arabinogalactans,* and *fructooligosaccharides* (FOS). Foods to focus on include the Microbiome Superfoods: asparagus, carrots, garlic, Jerusalem artichoke, jicama, leeks, okra, onion, radishes, and tomatoes, as well as the Microbiome Superspices, turmeric and cinnamon.

You will also reestablish intestinal balance with the correct ratio of Omega 3 to Omega 6 healthy fats by consuming nuts and nut butters (almond, macadamia, cashew), seeds and seed butters, flaxseed and flaxseed oil, sunflower seed oil, and olive oil. In addition, you will focus on high-quality proteins, high-fiber carbs, and lots of high-quality fresh fruits and vegetables. Finally, you will take probiotics, prebiotics, and the Microbiome Supersupplements needed to nourish your microbiome, heal your gut, and promote optimal health.

PHASE 2: THE METABOLIC BOOST

Support Your Microbiome to Boost Your Metabolism

In this phase you can eat a wider variety of foods, including eggs; sheep's and goat's milk yogurt and kefir (a yogurt-like drink made from fermented milk); and gluten-free whole grains such as buckwheat, brown rice, and wild rice. You continue to load up on the Microbiome Superfoods and Superspices and to take probiotics, prebiotics, and our Microbiome Supersupplements.

You also learn about the ways stress imbalances the microbiome, dramatically and quickly, within less than twenty-four hours. To help relieve stress I suggest brief meditations before each meal, techniques for focused eating, and approaches to creating each mealtime or snacktime as a brief but powerful moment to truly revel in the sensuous pleasures of eating.

PHASE 3: THE LIFETIME TUNE-UP

Maintaining Healthy Weight Loss for Life

In this final phase of the Microbiome Diet I establish basic parameters for supporting your microbiome and keeping your gut in good shape. I also explain that once your gut health has been restored, you only have to stick to this eating plan 70 percent of the time! You can add in some portions of the healthiest forms of gluten: whole-grain and sprouted breads and moderate amounts of barley, bulgur, wheat berries, and millet. And about 30 percent of the time you can indulge in most other foods, including the occasional sweet.

What I have found with my patients is that by the time they reach this phase of the eating plan they no longer suffer from food cravings, blood sugar spikes and crashes, or the other biological issues that cause so many people to break their diets and regain the weight they worked so hard to lose. Restoring their intestinal health and balancing the microbiome frees them from cravings and compulsions while putting them in touch with what their body needs and wants. It's almost as if they have awakened their "inner nutritionist," instinctively seeking the foods they need to remain healthy, energized, and fit.

Balancing your microbiome will also help you prevent or even reverse such conditions as rheumatoid arthritis, lupus, multiple sclerosis, and other autoimmune conditions. It works against headache, joint pain, sore muscles, and fatigue. A healthy microbiome even has some protective effects against cancer.

Another wonderful thing about the Microbiome Diet is the way it will transform your whole relationship to food, appetite, and perhaps even your own identity. Nourishing your microbiome will automatically free you from cravings, uncontrollable appetite, and the dispiriting feeling that your weight will stay on or return eventually no matter what you do. Instead, you'll feel empowered as well as newly connected to your own natural feelings of hunger and fullness.

As you become aware of the other ecology within your body, your view of your own identity may change as well. You will have the opportunity to experience a sense of connectedness to both the ecology within and the ecology without—a sense of how all creatures are profoundly connected to one another and to the planet.

But first things first. Here is a preview of the three phases of the Microbiome Diet, each of which is explained in detail in the next three sections of this book. As you can see, the entire diet is based on rebalancing your microbiome and healing your gut. Your metabolism will never be the same!

PART II

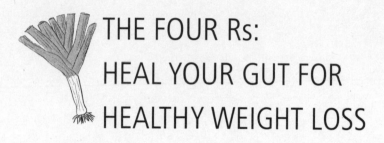

THE FOUR Rs:
HEAL YOUR GUT FOR
HEALTHY WEIGHT LOSS

three

REMOVE

THE FOUR Rs

▼ **Remove from the diet** anything that interferes with a healthy microbial balance or compromises intestinal health:

  ▶ Hydrochloric acid is crucial for digestion.

  ▶ Enzymes—protease, lipase, amylase, and DPP IV—help with the digestion of different types of food.

  ▶ No inflammatory, allergenic, or reactive foods: no sugar, eggs, soy, gluten, or dairy, and no products made with these foods

  ▶ No unhealthy fats: trans fats, hydrogenated fats

  ▶ No preservatives or additives

  ▶ No artificial sweeteners

  ▶ No environmental toxins

Remove from the gut parasites and the disproportionate growth of the wrong types of bacteria, known as *dysbiosis*, and break through the protective *biofilm* that protects yeast and the wrong types of bacteria, using the following natural compounds:

  ▶ Berberine, wormwood, caprylic acid, grapefruit seed extract, garlic, oregano oil

▷ Replace

▷ Reinoculate

▷ Repair

M Y PATIENT MARGO WAS FRUSTRATED. SHE DIDN'T UNDERSTAND why I seemed to be asking her to cut out so many "healthy choices" from her diet.

As I had explained to her, Phase 1 of the Microbiome Diet is my own adaptation of a protocol that functional medicine physicians use: the Four Rs. With this approach I would help Margo balance her microbiome and restore her intestinal health. We would be taking all four steps simultaneously over the three weeks of Phase 1.

I told Margo the "Remove" portion of this protocol had two aspects:

- **Remove from the diet** anything that interferes with a healthy microbial balance or compromises intestinal health.
- **Remove from the gut** parasites and the disproportionate growth of the wrong types of bacteria, known as *dysbiosis*, and break through the protective *biofilm* that protects yeast and the wrong types of bacteria.

Much of this protocol made sense to Margo. But when I started describing which foods she would have to avoid for the next three weeks, she balked.

"You want me to avoid eggs, soy, gluten, and dairy?" she said skeptically. "I've never heard of such a thing. Okay, maybe the gluten—I've heard about gluten-free and low-carb diets, and I can see why you wouldn't want me eating lots of bread. But I've never heard of a diet where you can't have egg whites! Or nonfat Greek yogurt! Or tofu! I can't believe those things are bad for you—*everybody* says they're healthy! And they don't have hardly any calories at all!"

I explained to Margo that we were not counting calories; we were looking at what kinds of food could rebalance her microbiome and support her intestinal health. That stubborn thirty pounds that Margo had not been able to lose since she had given birth to her first child told me she was almost certainly facing two problems: an imbalanced microbiome and a leaky gut. Both conditions were setting her up for inflammation and a fat-storing metabolism that clung to every ounce of fat for dear life.

Once you *rebalance your microbiome* and *repair your leaky gut* you can heal inflammation and reset your metabolism to burn fat rather than store it. This was my goal for Margo.

So on Phase 1 I wasn't concerned about counting calories or even about measuring fats and carbs; I was more concerned about making sure Margo avoided any foods that would feed her unhealthy bacteria and trigger a reaction from her immune system.

Phase 1 would go a long way toward rebalancing Margo's microbiome and healing her leaky gut, and this in turn would calm her immune system. As a result, by the time she reached Phase 2 Margo would be able to add moderate amounts of gluten-free whole grains to her diet: quinoa, brown rice, and spelt. Very likely she would be able to eat eggs too—not just the whites, but the whole egg, which is very healthy, especially when organic or free range. She might well be able to eat moderate amounts of dairy, especially goat's and sheep's milk products. And by the time she arrived at Phase 3 four weeks later her microbiome and her intestinal health would be in even better shape so at that point she might be able to eat the healthiest forms of gluten: whole-grain and sprouted breads and moderate amounts of barley, bulgur, wheat berries, and millet.

HOW "HEALTHY" BUT REACTIVE FOODS PROMOTE WEIGHT GAIN

Reactive foods leak through intestinal walls
⬇
Immune system goes on alert:
It makes antibodies and sends out
"killer chemicals"
⬇
Antibodies create cravings
⬇

Killer chemicals create inflammation
⬇
Inflammation leads to storing fat
instead of burning it

But before those foods would work for Margo, we had to rebalance her microbiome and restore gut health. That was why in Phase 1 I wanted Margo to cut out seemingly healthy foods: eggs, dairy, soy, gluten, and grains.

Margo was still having trouble with the idea of removing so many apparently healthy foods from her diet. So I broke it down for her, food by food.

REMOVE THE EGGS AND DAIRY

If you have been overweight for a while and, particularly, if you have struggled unsuccessfully to lose the weight, it is a good working assumption you have leaky gut and the system-wide inflammation that goes with it.

Assuming you do have leaky gut, your immune system is very likely overreacting to the partially digested foods that leak through your intestinal walls. Without testing, you cannot be sure exactly which foods are triggering a reaction. However, the most common reactive foods are eggs, dairy, soy, and gluten, so those are the four I would like you to cut out, at least for the first three weeks.

I explained to Margo that if her immune system was overreacting to dairy, even the tiniest amount—a spoonful of skim milk in her morning coffee or a sprinkling of cheese across her salad—would set off a significant immune reaction when it leaked through her intestinal walls.

Some immune reactions happened immediately and severely. Others, like many food sensitivities, are delayed for several hours or even a few days. This sometimes makes it difficult to link your symptoms to a food you eat, especially if you believe the food is healthy. But even if the symptoms are mild, the underlying immune reaction creates significant problems for your metabolism and your weight, especially if you keep triggering it by continuing to eat reactive foods.

So if Margo did have a tiny bit of dairy, eventually her immune system would zap the dairy molecules it detected, and Margo would develop symptoms, anything from acne to a sore throat to gas and bloating to aching joints. (For a more complete list of potential symptoms, see page 37. Those symptoms are both symptoms of an unbalanced microbiome and the signs of leaky gut, because almost always the two conditions go together.)

In addition Margo's system-wide inflammation would cue her pancreas to release excessive amounts of insulin, which would then cue her body to store fat instead of burn it. Thus, even a tiny amount of milk—insignificant in terms of calories or fat content but incredibly significant as an immune trigger—could make losing weight virtually impossible for Margo.

Likewise, even the minuscule amount of egg that might lurk in a salad dressing or a sauce would set Margo's alarm bells ringing. Her immune system would view the traces of egg as a "toxic invader," zapping it with powerful chemicals and creating the inflammatory cascade whose ultimate result is fat storage.

Once that immune reaction is in motion, all weight loss efforts are likely to be in vain. Even if you manage to take off a few pounds, they will almost certainly come back if you still have leaky gut and an overreactive immune system.

So before we could reintroduce eggs and dairy into Margo's diet we had to heal her leaky gut and reset her immune system. We had to take these foods completely out of her diet—even in the tiniest amounts—so there would not be even a single "anti-dairy" or "anti-egg" antibody left in her body.

At some point, I told Margo, she *would* be able to eat eggs and dairy again, especially sheep's and goat's milk dairy, which most people find easier to digest than cow's milk products. When Margo's leaky gut was healed, her immune system would very likely stop overreacting to these otherwise healthy choices. And if we kept these foods out of her system long enough, her immune system would eventually stop making the antibodies to them. No more immune reactions, no more inflammation, and no more excessive fat storage.

And, as an added bonus, no more cravings. Without the egg-and-dairy-seeking antibodies triggered by her immune system, Margo could stop feeling as though she was addicted to those types of foods.

A balanced microbiome and a healthy immune system also meant Margo's ghrelin (the hormone regulating hunger) and leptin (the hormone regulating fullness) would return to a healthy balance. As a result Margo would feel hungry only when she really needed nourishment and would feel full after she had eaten the food her body required. Finally, she could stop feeling like her appetite was raging out of control.

REMOVE THE SOY

Soy, I explained to Margo, was another common trigger for immune system reactions and leaky gut. But even when Margo's system had healed I didn't want her eating large amounts of soy, which tends to imbalance thyroid levels and has unpredictable effects on estrogen.

Once Margo's immune system and leaky gut were fully healed she might no longer be sensitive to soy. But because of its potential effects on her thyroid hormone levels, I still wanted her to leave it out of her diet.

By the way, processed soy is added to a surprisingly wide variety of foods because it is such an effective preservative. You can find it in chocolate, cereals, fast food hamburgers, and a wide variety of baked goods and other commercial food products. So another danger of eating processed foods is that doing so loads your body up with far too much soy.

REMOVE THE GLUTEN

Gluten, I told Margo, posed a slightly different type of challenge to her system. But again, my concern wasn't about the calories but rather the chemistry.

Gluten is a form of protein found in wheat, barley, rye, and other grains. It is also used as a preservative so frequently you can almost always find it in any type of baked good or processed food, including ketchup, soy sauce, salad dressings, gravies, canned soup, processed meats, and cold cuts. Just about any reduced-fat product contains gluten to make the product gel better, including low-fat ice cream. Manufacturers generally add significant amounts of gluten to ready-made meals, frozen dinners, and fast foods because of gluten's ability to extend these products' shelf life. You can also find gluten in personal care products, such as toothpaste, shampoo, and body lotion, and these significantly increase your exposure to it, whether you are absorbing it through your gut, the mucous membranes in your mouth, or the pores of your skin.

We all react to gluten in different ways. About 1 percent of the population has an extreme reaction to gluten known as celiac disease. If Margo had been in that 1 percent, I would have told her she simply had to avoid gluten in all its forms, even in the tiniest amounts, for the rest of her life. If you think you have celiac disease, I urge you to visit your health care provider and get tested for this condition.

Yet even people who don't have celiac can be sensitive to gluten, just as they can be sensitive to eggs, dairy, and soy. That's because gluten triggers the production of *zonulin*. Zonulin is a biochemical that opens up the tight junctions of your intestinal wall. When you eat gluten in moderate amounts—say, a twice-weekly serving of toast or pasta—your body has a chance to tighten up those junctions and maintain intestinal health. But when you are continually exposed to gluten, not only in breads and pastas but also in all the processed foods, food products, and personal care products that contain it, your tight junctions often remain open, causing you to develop leaky gut.

As a result gluten can leak into your system, setting off an immune reaction, causing your system to develop antigluten antibodies, and putting you in a constant state of low-grade inflammation. And, as you recall, inflammation almost always leads to weight gain.

As you can see, my concern has more to do with an immune system reaction than with calories or even carbs. That's why restricting gluten isn't enough in the first phase of the Microbiome Diet—you have to cut it out entirely. You're not lowering your caloric intake or your carb consumption; you are freeing your body from an immune system trigger. For your immune system to calm down and stop over-reacting, it has to be given a complete rest.

So, I told Margo, we would begin the Microbiome Diet by eliminating gluten entirely, and we would avoid gluten through both Phase 1 and Phase 2. By Phase 3, however, Margo might be able to introduce small amounts of gluten back into her diet because at that point her immune system and her intestinal health would be sufficiently restored, partly because her newly balanced microbiome would also be giving her whole system additional support. If you have good intestinal and microbial health, you can safely consume gluten two or three times a week, although if you suffer from an autoimmune condition or are inclined to anxiety or depression, you should avoid gluten altogether.

REMOVE THE GRAINS

In most people gluten-free grains—quinoa, brown rice, and spelt—are unlikely to set off food sensitivities. Even when these grains leak through our intestinal walls, most immune systems do not react. But as we saw in Chapter 2, bad bacteria love the sugars and starches found in grains, even whole grains. And I didn't want Margo eating anything that would feed the bad bacteria—I wanted to starve them out.

By the time Margo got to Phase 2 her microbiome would be far more balanced, with a flourishing population of good bacteria. At that point eating whole grains would nourish those good bacteria, which would benefit from the fiber and other nutrients.

Now, however, Margo was just starting Phase 1, and her microbiome was still loaded with bad bacteria. Those bacteria would benefit far too much even from whole grains, and Margo could get fiber and nutrients from our Microbiome Superfoods instead. Best to avoid the grains in Phase 1 and let the rebalancing begin!

REMOVE THE SUGAR

Margo understood in a general way why sugar was not a healthy choice for dieters. But I wanted her to see this decision in terms of chemistry, not calories.

There are two major problems with sugar for anyone who is trying to lose weight. One is that sugar acts very quickly to send your blood sugar spiking, which triggers a flood of insulin. As we have seen, excess insulin sets you up for insulin resistance and also cues your body for fat storage.

The other problem with sugar is how well it nourishes the disruptive bacteria in your microbiome. When you have reached Phase 3 of the Microbiome Diet you can maintain only 70 percent compliance and indulge occasionally in moderate amounts of sugar — say, a dessert once or twice a week. But while you are trying to rebalance your microbiome and reset your metabolism avoid sweets and refined flour so you aren't inadvertently feeding the bad bacteria.

REMOVE ARTIFICIAL SWEETENERS

If I had to pick my top ten myths about diet and health, the idea that artificial sweeteners are a good substitute for sugar would surely be on that list. Artificial sweeteners create numerous problems for your health *and* for your weight. Aspartame (sold as Nutrasweet and Equal) breaks down into such harmful compounds as formaldehyde, which is highly likely to cause cancer. Some research has associated sucralose (sold as Splenda) with leukemia.

In addition, sucralose can cause your blood sugar levels to spike and your insulin to spike as well, putting you at risk for both insulin resistance and weight gain. And all artificial sweeteners can cause *calorie dysregulation*. Our bodies are initially programmed to associate sweetness with a high amount of calories and, therefore, to become "full" quickly when eating sweet foods. Eating sweet no-calorie foods teaches our bodies to break that connection, which can cause us to remain hungry even after consuming lots of calories.

Researchers have therefore implicated artificial sweeteners in weight gain, increased hunger, cravings, and even depression. In September 2013 a review of the scientific literature published in *Obesity Reviews* showed that sugar substitutes also have an impact on the microbiome, which might well be why they have had those other negative effects.

You can see why I would like you to permanently avoid all artificial sweeteners! However, Lakanto, made from a sugar alcohol and calorie-free, is a healthy substitute in moderation. It does not raise your glucose or your insulin levels. It's granulated, so you can use it to sweeten your coffee or tea or to cook and bake with. You can easily find Lakanto online for purchase.

REMOVE UNHEALTHY FATS

One of the best things you can do for your microbiome and your digestion is to remove unhealthy fats from your diet. By unhealthy fats, I mean particularly *trans fats* and *hydrogenated fats*.

Basically these two forms of fats were invented to extend food products' shelf life. They are not natural foods, and they did not co-evolve with us *or* our microbiome. They are incompatible with our physiology, wreak havoc on our digestive enzymes, and promote inflammation, which, as we have seen, can lead to weight gain. These unnatural fats can also lead to the production of free radicals, which destroy the health of your cells.

To understand the true damage these fats wreak, remember that every single cell in your body is surrounded by a *membrane*, a cell wall, charged with two important jobs. On the one hand, your cell walls must allow for the free movement of nutrients into the cell so the cell is nourished. On the other hand, they must prevent toxins from entering the cell so the cell is protected.

Because your cell walls are made of fat, they need healthy fats to do their jobs. So when you consume trans or hydrogenated fats you no longer have a healthy cell wall regulating what gets into and out of your cells. Nor do you have optimal digestion, energy burning, or fat burning.

On an even deeper level, whatever enters your cells affects your DNA, the genetic acids that help determine who you are. Unhealthy cell membranes expose your DNA to the wrong types of influences, undermining your health and setting you up for the worst rather than the best version of your genetic inheritance.

As we saw in Chapter 2, unhealthy fats also feed the wrong types of bacteria, the disruptive microbes that produce endotoxins, spark inflammation, and cue your body to store fat. Eating unhealthy fats can almost instantly disrupt your microbiome and put you on the road to weight gain.

The good news is that loading your diet up with healthy fats will keep your cell walls in optimal condition. The right balance of Omega 3s (found in fish oil, flaxseed oil, nuts, and seeds) and Omega 6s (the healthiest forms of which are found in olive oil and avocado) will help. In Phases 1 and 2 of the Microbiome Diet you practice loading up your diet with healthy fats so by the time you are creating your own meal plans in Phase 3 you will be used to eating in a way that keeps your cells in peak condition.

REMOVE ADDITIVES AND PRESERVATIVES

Gluten is one major additive/preservative found throughout processed foods. Another is high-fructose corn syrup, a dangerous sweetener that feeds unhealthy bacteria, disrupts your hormones for hunger and fullness, and blunts your appetite for healthier foods.

Other chemical additives and preservatives extend the shelf life of your food and might enhance its color, flavor, or texture, but they also stress your liver, which must filter them out of your bloodstream, and this makes your liver less efficient at metabolizing fat. Although extensive research has not yet been done, I suspect these unnatural components of our food supply also disrupt our microbiome.

REMOVE DISRUPTIVE BACTERIA

If you are overweight and especially if you have been struggling to lose that weight, your current microbiome is not your friend. Regardless of any diet you might go on, the microbiome presently living in your body is determined to make you store fat. Sure, you can restrict calories, cut back on refined carbs, avoid sugar, or make some other potentially healthy change, and your microbiome might play along with you for a few weeks or even a few months. But ultimately it knows it's going to win, cuing you to be hungry all the time, to overeat, and to feed it with the greasy, starchy, sugary diet that it craves.

Unhealthy levels of insulin, blood sugar, leptin, and ghrelin—levels determined by an unhealthy microbiome—are why so many dieters feel hungry and unsatisfied with their supposedly healthy diets and why they so often gain back all the weight they lost. In order to achieve a permanently healthy weight you have to *remove* the disruptive bacteria that have hijacked your microbiome.

I'll give you one quick example of how dramatically bad bacteria can disrupt your microbiome to create weight gain. Researchers in Shanghai studied mice that were actually bred to resist obesity. These mice stayed slim even when they were fed a high-calorie diet. They had the type of genes that most of us would envy.

Yet when these genetically slim mice were injected with bacteria known as *enterobacter*, a microbe frequently found in overweight humans, they gained weight. The enterobacter was more powerful than the "slender" genes.

I must admit that I was particularly excited to read this study because I myself had been aware of the dangers of the enterobacter. I had given many of my overweight patients stool tests to see whether this microbe had colonized them, and for most of them the answer was yes. When I removed the bug from their system they began immediately to lose weight.

The Shanghai researchers confirmed my observation. One of them commented that enterobacter "may causatively contribute to the development of obesity in humans."

REMOVE FUNGI, PARASITES, AND YEAST

Both fungi and parasites disrupt your digestion and might well imbalance your microbiome as well. When you have too much yeast in
your microbiome it also becomes imbalanced, and you tend to crave
sugar and starches as a result.

One common example of this is the condition known as candida
albicans, which is associated with numerous symptoms both inside
and outside the gut: intestinal bloating, gas, constipation, diarrhea,
and abdominal discomfort as well as skin rashes, vaginal yeast, fatigue, brain fog, anxiety, depression, muscle and joint pain, excessive
hunger, and cravings for sweets, just to name a few.

Parasites are quite common and, unfortunately, frequently difficult to diagnose by stool testing. They too can lead to symptoms similar to those caused by candida.

Frequently, people who suffer from autoimmune conditions also
suffer from candida and/or parasites. Fortunately, whatever the diagnosis, the solution is the same: break through the biofilm that protects the
yeast and use natural compounds to remove parasites. To accomplish
all these tasks I suggest you use the following natural compounds:
berberine, wormwood, caprylic acid, grapefruit seed extract, garlic,
oregano oil.

You'll find more detail about our Microbiome Supersupplements
in the section on Microbiome Superfoods (page 161).

REMOVE ENVIRONMENTAL TOXINS

Environmental toxins have so many interrelated effects on your
body that it's hard to know where to start. Here's a partial list. Environmental toxins

- Disrupt your endocrine system—your hormones—and this
  can affect your metabolism and weight;
- Create inflammation as they stress your immune system,
  which, again, can affect metabolism and weight; and

- Stress your liver—your major detox organ—which must filter them out of your blood, and this means your liver is likely to metabolize fat less efficiently, again affecting metabolism and weight.

Although little research has been done on how environmental toxins affect your microbiome, it stands to reason that the microbial life within your intestines responds differently to toxins, heavy metals, and genetically modified crops than it does to the unadulterated food, water, and air that existed on our planet for the last several million years. We do know environmental toxins set you up for inflammation and, potentially, autoimmune disorders such as rheumatoid arthritis, multiple sclerosis, lupus, and fibromyalgia. So very likely they disrupt your microbiome while they are also wreaking havoc on your immune system.

There are two ways you can defend against environmental toxins. One is to make every effort to eat organic, drink filtered water, avoid polluted air, and use household and cosmetic products that do not contain toxic chemicals. I advise you to make your best efforts, but realistically, until we humans collectively decide to clean up our planet's ecology, there is only so much that you, individually, can do.

Your other recourse is to improve your inner ecology, making it as robust and healthy as possible so you have the best possible defense against anything coming at you from outside. Supporting your microbiome and your intestinal health through the Four Rs protocol in Phase 1 is an excellent place to start.

REMOVE CALORIE COUNTING AND GUILT

One of the most exciting breakthroughs in microbiome science is the way it transforms our whole relationship to weight loss and obesity. Learning about the microbiome idea is a real paradigm shifter, offering us the opportunity to remove the misconceptions, misguided ideas, and toxic notions so many of us have about food and dieting.

REMOVE, AS MUCH AS POSSIBLE, THESE DANGERS TO YOUR MICROBIOME

- Additives and preservatives.
- Antibiotics—obviously sometimes they are vital to your health, but avoid overuse and always take probiotics when you are taking antibiotics.
- Chlorine.
- Environmental toxins.
- Excessive and unremitting stress.
- Genetically modified organisms (GMOs).
- Hand sanitizers, except when absolutely necessary— your body needs to be exposed to more bacteria.
- Heavy metals, such as the mercury found in many large fish. For updated information on which fish are safest to eat, visit the following website: http://epi.publichealth .nc.gov/oee/mercury/safefish.html.
- Meat from animals treated inhumanely or raised inorganically—they feed on genetically modified feed, and are full of stress chemicals from their inhumane treatment. Until recently they have been loaded with antibiotics, and even after new FDA regulations go into effect, they will still be a significant source of antibiotics in our diet. After all, 80 percent of all antibiotics in this country are consumed in our food, so the FDA restrictions are unlikely to solve the problem.
- NSAIDS—nonsteroidal anti-inflammatory drugs, including aspirin and ibuprofen—except when absolutely necessary. Despite the fact that they reduce inflammation, they also damage the sensitive mucosal lining of the gut and, therefore, hurt the microbiome, leading ultimately to more inflammation and, eventually, weight gain.
- Processed foods.
- Sugar and refined carbohydrates.
- Trans fats and hydrogenated fats.

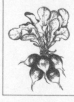

So many of my patients come to me with guilt and shame about their previous inability to lose weight or their yo-yo dieting. They see their experience as a failure of will or as evidence they are lazy, greedy, gluttonous, or somehow inferior to the thin people they know, especially the ones who seem to be able to indulge in a slice of pizza or a rich dessert and somehow still remain slender.

I want them—and you—to understand this guilt is misplaced. Your microbiome is more powerful than you, and the inflammatory process it ignites has powerful consequences for your metabolism and your weight as well as your energy levels, focus, concentration, and mood. Fatigue, brain fog, anxiety, and depression so often accompany an imbalanced microbiome and an inflamed digestive system, and these, too, are not your fault. They are the inevitable by-products of your system going out of balance. Rebalance your biology, and many of these problems will disappear. If you do need to make changes in your life, this revitalization will give you the energy, motivation, and self-confidence to do so.

It's hard to grasp how profoundly your biology has you in its grasp, especially when you feel anxious, depressed, or exhausted. But once you have completed Phase 1 of the Microbiome Diet you will be astonished at how different you feel simply because your entire body chemistry has begun to shift.

So remove the idea that you're to blame for what is happening with your body—that only creates a downward spiral of guilt and shame that makes you feel even worse, saps more of your energy, and makes genuine change seem even further out of reach. Remove from your thoughts the dietary advice that comes from other people, trust your own gut reactions, and let your inner ecology speak to you.

four

REPLACE

Z OE WAS A TALL, STRIKING WOMAN IN HER FIFTIES WHO HAD BEEN fighting "that extra ten pounds" for years. Since she had gone into menopause, she told me bluntly, "everything just went completely to hell," and she had picked up another fifteen pounds.

"I see myself just getting heavier and heavier," she told me, "and I'm worried it's just going to *keep* getting worse and worse and worse. I haven't really changed my diet, but suddenly my metabolism is just

71

out of control. I've tried to exercise more, but it just makes me hungrier. Nobody believes me, Dr. Kellman! They're all sure I've started bingeing or slacking off on my workouts, but I really haven't changed anything, and yet I just keep gaining weight."

I reassured Zoe that *I* believed her. I had seen hundreds of patients over the years who had described the exact same story to me. Suddenly—perhaps after childbirth, a course of antibiotics, or menopause or andropause (a hormonal shift in aging men)—the eating habits that had worked for a lifetime had suddenly stopped working. In many cases the person had been slightly overweight before but now were gaining much more weight, more quickly, and they didn't know how to make it stop. Often, as was also true with Zoe, their previous pattern had been to gain a little extra weight, diet and exercise intensively, lose the extra weight, and be fine for a while before they began to gain some weight again. Then, at some point, they became unable to lose the extra weight even as they began gaining more and more.

Zoe breathed out a sign of relief as I told her she was not alone. The feeling that your metabolism has been hijacked is an extremely common one. When your microbiome goes out of balance and cues an alteration in your metabolism, there *is* another force affecting the way you relate to food. Your levels of leptin and ghrelin, the hormones that regulate fullness and hunger, go out of balance as well, so your appetite as well as your metabolism seems to be in the grip of an alien force.

I asked Zoe to describe what happened during and after a typical meal. As we talked, Zoe began to realize that for quite some time she had been having digestive symptoms she simply hadn't associated with her weight problem. She told me her stomach often felt very full after a meal, as though the food was staying in it for too long. She also described frequent gas and bloating about three or four hours after she ate.

I explained to Zoe that these problems were likely because of a lack of digestive enzymes and stomach acid. We need stomach acid to break down our food so it can be passed into the small intestine.

There, digestive enzymes break the food down further into components small enough to be absorbed.

Most people, I told Zoe, are not digesting their food properly because of a shortage of enzymes, acids, or both. That shortage contributes to leaky gut and also stresses your digestive system.

That is why the second component of the Four Rs protocol for gut health is *Replace*: replace the enzymes and stomach acid you need for optimal digestion. Luckily this is fairly easy to do. As you'll see in the food plan for Phase 1 on page 185, you simply take digestive enzymes with every meal and snack as well as hydrochloric acid tablets to help you supplement your stomach acid.

Zoe understood immediately why the enzymes were important. But she was confused about taking stomach acid because, it turned out, her doctor had put her on Prilosec, a proton pump inhibitor intended to reduce stomach acid.

"Why on earth would I need more?" she asked me. "I had a lot of heartburn before I started taking the Prilosec—now I'm fine!"

"Maybe you don't have heartburn at the moment," I replied. "But the proton pump inhibitor is actually making your digestion worse. It might even be related to your weight gain."

Zoe was more confused than ever, so I gave her a full explanation.

REPLACE: STOMACH ACID

When you swallow some food, it passes from your mouth down through your esophagus to your stomach. There, your stomach secretes hydrochloric acid to dissolve the proteins in your food. Your stomach also secretes *pepsin*, a digestive enzyme that further helps with digestion.

But when your stomach isn't producing enough acid this portion of the digestive process breaks down. And it is a very significant breakdown. Reduced levels of stomach acid can impair the absorption of nutrients as well as B6, folate (another crucial form of vitamin B), calcium, and iron. Insufficient stomach acid also predisposes us to *dysbiosis*, the imbalance of bacteria in the microbiome.

In fact, paradoxically, low stomach acid is often the cause of heartburn. That unpleasant burning sensation after a meal is not caused by too much acid but rather by too little.

How can this be? Well, that burning sensation is caused by acid reflux, also known as GERD, gastroesophageal reflux disorder. When your stomach acid is low, your food isn't moving through your system at the proper speed, hence that feeling of "extra fullness." Instead of being propelled forward into the small intestine, the contents of your stomach reflux back up into the esophagus along with some acid, which tends to burn. The solution is not to reduce the acid further but to increase it so your system pushes the food forward instead of refluxing it back.

Burning does not always indicate insufficient acid. Some people *do* have excess acid, and heartburn is their symptom as well. For the vast majority of people, however, heartburn and acid reflux are indicators of insufficient stomach acid. In Phase 1 of the Microbiome Diet I explain how to replace your stomach acid—naturally.

REMOVE: PROTON PUMP INHIBITORS

Now at this point you might be wondering, if low stomach acid causes heartburn, why do acid-reducing medications like antacids and

	SIGNS OF LOW STOMACH ACID
belching	nausea after taking supplements
bloating	
burning	rosacea, indicated by dilated blood vessels in the nose or cheeks
constipation	
excessive gas in upper part of intestine	sense of excessive fullness after eating, as though your food is just sitting in your stomach and not being digested
flatulence immediately after meals	
food allergies	
indigestion	

proton pump inhibitors make the burning stop? The answer is that
the meds *do* stop the burning from the acids that have refluxed back
into your esophagus because they reduce *that* acid. But by reducing
the acids they are also impairing your digestion. In my view it's a little
like trying to stop a headache by cutting off the person's head—yes,
the pain will stop, but there are likely to be other problems!

In fact, one of the reasons our microbiomes are in such distress
is because of the widespread overuse of antacids and proton pump
inhibitors. The makers of these products have put on an amazing
marketing campaign, and they have had incredible success in selling
their wares. But they have not succeeded in improving our overall
health—rather, the opposite. Some people do occasionally need relief from heartburn or acid reflux, and these medications may be war-
ranted in the short term. In the long term, however, these products
compromise the microbiome as well as the entire digestive process.

It's not just about digestion. Hydrochloric acid also works to keep
unfriendly bacteria and yeast out of your system. So if you don't have
enough hydrochloric acid, you throw your microbiome even further
off balance. Perhaps this is why the use of proton pump inhibitors
has been associated with increased allergies and infections, including pneumonia:

imbalanced microbiome	**+**	compromised digestion	**=**	immune difficulties, other symptoms, weight gain

As if this weren't bad enough, a December 2013 article published
by the *Journal of the American Medical Association,* based on a huge
study of more than twenty-five thousand patients, found that people
taking proton pump inhibitors for more than two years are 65 percent more likely to suffer from a vitamin B12 deficiency. The association was strongest in patients under the age of thirty. A deficit in
vitamin B12 has been associated with anemia, fatigue, memory loss,
brain fog, and other brain dysfunctions.

So taking regular antacids or relying long term on a proton pump
inhibitor could be setting you up for significant problems. Cut out

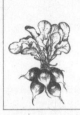

Causes of Low Stomach Acid
alcohol
antibiotics, which imbalance the microbiome
caffeine
hypothyroidism
imbalanced microbiome—especially the lack of *h. pylori*
nicotine
stress, especially chronic stress

these meds and follow the protocol I offer in Phase 1 to replace your stomach acid naturally. (Check with your physician before cutting out any prescription medications, including a proton pump inhibitor.)

REPLACE: ENZYMES

Once your food passes from the stomach to the small intestine, digestive enzymes begin to break it down further so its nutrients can be absorbed into the bloodstream. However, insufficient stomach acid means the small intestine never gets the full signal to produce those enzymes, and this is another reason you probably need both extra hydrochloric acid and supplemental enzymes.

Now, guess what else stimulates the small intestine to produce digestive enzymes? If you guessed "your microbiome," you are correct. But when your microbiome is unhealthy or unbalanced it does not give this crucial signal. As a result your digestion is compromised. You don't get the full nutritional value of the food you eat, and if you have leaky gut, your partially digested food is more likely to cross the intestinal wall, setting off yet another inflammatory immune response.

When I explained this whole process to Zoe, she understood why insufficient stomach acid as well as depleted enzymes might be at work in her weight loss difficulties. She embarked on the protocol I lay out on page 73 to replace both stomach acid and enzymes along with the rest of the Phase 1 program. To her surprise, she noticed an immediate difference in how she felt after eating, even though she had not really been aware of digestive issues before. Her experience was similar to that of many of my patients. Sometimes things have to improve before you realize how bad they were!

REPLACE: YOUR ATTITUDE TOWARD FOOD

In the previous chapter I asked you to remove calorie counting and guilt from your approach to weight loss. In this chapter I'd like you to consider replacing your old approach to food. Instead of viewing food as your enemy, I'd like you to cultivate a deep appreciation and gratitude for the wonderful experience of eating.

After all, food is one of the great pleasures of life. Think of how satisfying it is to bite into a crisp, tangy apple; to savor a delicious, lemony piece of broiled fish; to linger over the last few sips of a fragrant cup of tea or a well-brewed cup of coffee. Recall how delightful it is to join your friends for a meal, how romantic to share an intimate dinner with a new love, how deeply bonding it can be to prepare dinner with your family. At its most primal level food is our basic connection to the planet.

We'll talk more about focused, appreciative eating in Part III. But meanwhile, if you're tempted to think of food as the enemy, to count every bite you put into your mouth, or to think of food restriction as "being good" and indulging as "being bad," I invite you to replace that attitude. The more you enjoy your food and the more you appreciate the bounty of our planet, the more you are likely to make truly healthy, nourishing food choices. After years of treating overweight patients, I have come to believe that eating on the run or in stressful, unsatisfying circumstances plays a significant role in weight gain, while eating in a focused, appreciative, satisfying way can make a huge difference in weight loss. So while you are replacing missing enzymes and stomach acids, replace your missing enjoyment and appreciation as well.

five

REINOCULATE

The Four Rs

▷ Remove

▷ Replace

▼ **Reinoculate yourself with:**

- ▸ **Probiotics**—the friendly bacteria that populate the gut. You can take them in capsule form or by eating cultured and fermented foods that contain live bacteria: raw sauerkraut, kimchee, and fermented vegetables throughout the Microbiome Diet; goat's or sheep's milk kefir and yogurt in Phases 2 and 3.

- ▸ **Prebiotics**—the foods and supplements that help friendly bacteria to flourish. You can take prebiotics in capsule form or by eating Microbiome Superfoods rich in fiber: asparagus, carrots, garlic, Jerusalem artichoke, jicama, leeks, onions, radishes, and tomato.

▷ Reinoculate

▷ Repair

TARA, THE CREATIVE DIRECTOR AT AN ADVERTISING AGENCY, HAD always tried to eat healthy and stay fit. In her image-oriented profession she felt looking good was important, especially as her company dealt with so many clients in fashion and media. Surrounded by slender actresses and rail-thin models, Tara had always felt somewhat self-conscious about her body, but she knew she had a healthy weight, a stylish wardrobe, and loads of focused energy.

Then, after a visit home for Thanksgiving, Tara picked up an ear infection from her favorite niece. With the help of antibiotics Tara quickly recovered and thought no more about it—until, much to her dismay, she began to gain weight.

The practitioner who prescribed the antibiotics did not believe Tara's claim that the meds had somehow caused her weight gain. He insisted that she must have begun eating more or exercising less. Tara went to two or three other physicians for help with her mysterious weight problem, but none of them were inclined to credit the idea that antibiotics had played a role, and none of them had any suggestions beyond, "eat less," "exercise more," and "maybe try one of those diet programs with the support groups or the prepackaged meals." Because she seemed so upset about her weight, one of the doctors offered Tara antidepressants.

In despair, Tara came to me. By this point she was not only concerned about her weight gain but also about some other symptoms: brain fog, lack of energy, and trouble falling asleep. "I've never had any of these kinds of problems before," she told me. "I feel like I'm going crazy!"

I reassured Tara she was not going crazy; rather, she was suffering from the disruptive effect of antibiotics on her microbiome. After all, antibiotics are designed to kill microbes, but they are often not able to target *which* microbes to kill—the unfriendly ones that caused Tara's ear infection or the friendly ones that kept Tara's weight in balance, gave her energy, and kept her feeling sharp and focused.

I told Tara that not only had many of my other patients shared her experience but there was also a huge amount of scientific research to support the relationship of antibiotics and weight gain. We also know that farmers have deliberately used those meds to pack more pounds onto their cows, pigs, chickens, and turkeys, so clearly, there is a link! I reassured Tara that we could easily correct the problem

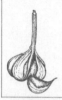

IF YOU MUST TAKE ANTIBIOTICS . . .

Sometimes, antibiotics are a necessary and very welcome response to an illness. But they can also significantly disrupt your microbiome. If you need to take antibiotics, be sure to also follow my recommendations for probiotics and prebiotics, on page 79. You should do this regardless of whether you want to lose weight, because otherwise the antibiotics might cause you to *gain* weight as well as potentially undermine your health in other ways.

with the Microbiome Diet, where, in Phase 1, we reinoculate with *probiotics* and *prebiotics*.

Tara was excited to think she could restore her previous healthy weight as well her former energy, clarity, and sharpness. Most of all, she was relieved to know something really had gone wrong with her metabolism, something that could definitely be fixed.

"Knowing that there's a good reason to follow this diet will help me stick to it," she told me. "From what you tell me, my microbiome was in good shape most of my life, but then it went out of whack. Believe me, I never want to go through that again!"

REINOCULATE TO CREATE DIVERSITY

In the last few years scientists have come to realize the overwhelming importance of diversity. Biodiversity, the presence of many different kinds of life, seems to be crucial to the health of any ecosystem, and the microbiome is no different. The more different species of bacteria that your microbiome contains, the healthier you are likely to be.

Part of the reason diversity matters is because your microbiome performs so many different tasks. A diverse microbiome is more likely to have enough of the right types of bacteria to do each of their jobs well. As you move through life, encountering a wide variety of different environments—and different diets—a diverse microbiome is far better equipped to protect you against any new threats that might arise, to get the most nutrients out of any food source, and to cope generally with new conditions.

A key function of the microbiome is to protect you against *pathogens*: a bacterium, fungus, or virus that might otherwise cause you harm. So a diverse microbiome is able to protect you against a wider variety of such dangers.

For example, *Lactobacillus casei gg*, a microbe the dairy industry uses to ripen cheddar cheese, also makes a compound that protects you from a variety of gastrointestinal diseases. If patients with Crohn's disease are given this type of bacteria, their immune function improves.

Another type of this bacteria, known as *Lactobacillus plant strain Number 14*, has been shown to reduce the size of fat cells. It also causes you to lose weight.

A different species, the *Bifidobacterium*, also seems to protect against gut infection as well as help to improve and modulate immune response through a wide variety of mechanisms. They also help to prevent enzymatic activity that might lead to cancer. *Bifidobacteria* also help your system produce vitamins.

Here are just a few of the other tasks various species perform within your microbiome:

- Producing short-chain fatty acids (SCFAs), which, as we have seen, are necessary for intestinal health, combat inflammation, and promote weight loss. SCFAs also help protect against colon cancer.
- Improving the health and strength of gut walls, helping to prevent leaky gut and, thereby, helping to prevent inflammation. This ultimately helps prevent unhealthy weight gain and contributes to the maintenance of a healthy weight.
- Maintaining the "tight junctions" between the cells in the lining of your intestinal walls, thereby preventing leaky gut.
- Improving nutrient absorption.
- Breaking down toxins.

- Preventing or easing autoimmune disorders, such as rheumatoid arthritis, lupus, and multiple sclerosis.

As a physician, I am especially interested in that last point, because I know conventional approaches to combat autoimmune disorders are so problematic. People with autoimmune conditions are typically prescribed strong drugs to suppress or modulate their immune system, drugs that often have limited effectiveness and serious side effects. I am thrilled to imagine that instead of depending on a pharmaceutical company's imperfect efforts to cure a disease, we can rely upon the ancient wisdom of nature itself to help us balance our systems and, thereby, restore them to health.

REINOCULATE TO ACHIEVE AND MAINTAIN A HEALTHY WEIGHT

As we saw in Chapter 2, numerous studies have demonstrated that when subjects are given probiotics, they lose both pounds and inches as body fat melts away. Significantly, the fat lost tends to be *visceral fat*, the highly dangerous fat wrapped around your organs that makes your abdomen bulge.

Visceral fat is not only unsightly; it's also unhealthy. When inflammation cues your body to hold onto visceral fat, it also sets off a truly vicious cycle:

inflammation
⬇
visceral fat
⬇
more inflammation
⬇
leaky gut
⬇
disrupted microbiome
⬇
more inflammation
⬇
more visceral fat

Losing that visceral fat, which probiotics has been shown to help you do, is the best, healthiest, and most attractive type of weight loss. And it turns that vicious cycle into a "virtuous cycle":

probiotics
⬇
balanced microbiome
⬇
reduced inflammation
⬇
loss of visceral fat
⬇
reduced inflammation
⬇
healthier microbiome
⬇
rebalanced immune system and metabolism
⬇
a body cued to maintain a healthy weight

REINOCULATE WITH FERMENTED FOODS

Fermented foods, such as sauerkraut, kimchee, fermented vegetables, yogurt, and kefir, are natural probiotics. They contain their own living cultures of bacteria, which supplement the healthy bacteria in your microbiome.

Because fermented foods are such a great way to replenish the bacteria in your microbiome, I have included several servings of kimchee, sauerkraut, and fermented vegetables throughout the Microbiome Diet in addition to having you take probiotics in pill form, and in Phase 2 I add several dishes prepared with kefir or yogurt.

I find it significant that just about every culture around the world has its own way of preparing fermented foods. To me, this near-universal recognition indicates how important this natural probiotic is to support our health. You can read more about fermented foods in Chapter 11, Your Microbiome Superfoods.

WHAT KINDS OF PROBIOTICS DO WE NEED?

- *Acidophilus reuteri*
- *Bifidobacter*
- *Bifidobacterium bifidus*
- *Bifidobacterium breve*
- *Bifidobacterium lactis*
- *Bifidobacterium longum*
- *Lactobacillus acidophilus*
- *Lactobacillus acidophilus*

- *Lactobacillus bulgaricus*
- *Lactobacillus casei gg*
- *Lactobacillus sporogenes*
- *Lactobacillus thermophiles*
- L N C F M
- *Plantarum*
- *Sachromyces boulardii*

For more information on choosing a probiotic supplement, see page 163.

REINOCULATE WITH PREBIOTICS

There's been a lot of talk about probiotics, but what about prebiotics? As we have seen, probiotics are the living bacteria that replenish our microbiome. You can find natural probiotics in fermented foods, such as sauerkraut, kimchee, fermented vegetables, yogurt, and kefir, or you can consume them in the form of pills. Prebiotics, by contrast, are the foods that feed our healthy bacteria: plant fibers found in our Microbiome Superfoods, such as asparagus, carrots, Jerusalem artichoke, jicama, leeks, onions, radishes, and tomatoes.

I actually prefer prebiotics to probiotics because with them we nourish the friendly bacteria that are already present. When you want to restock a polluted lake with fish, you don't just dump in new fish; you also clean up the lake, and then, almost spontaneously, the fish population will begin to flourish.

Prebiotics can be effective in producing weight loss and have always been shown to help prevent and even reverse nonalcoholic fatty liver disease, the condition that occurs when excess fat is stored in your liver. This is important for weight loss, as a liver weighed down by fat cannot help you lose weight.

What Kinds of Prebiotics Do We Need?

Here is a brief list of some key prebiotics:

- Arabinogalactans, found in carrots, kiwi, radishes, and tomatoes as well as the bark of the larch tree
- Inulin, found in, garlic, Jerusalem artichoke, jicama, and onions

Furthermore, prebiotics help overcome insulin resistance, which, as we shall see in later chapters, directly contributes to weight gain. Finally, people who take prebiotics have slimmer waists and a lower body mass index (BMI), meaning they have less fat proportional to the rest of their bodies as well as slimmed waists.

REINOCULATE YOURSELF WITH CONNECTION

Most diet books talk only about what to eat. But I also want you to think about *why* you are eating and *how* you are eating. After all, your relationship to food is a crucial aspect of your relationship to life. The two are profoundly interconnected; in fact, your emotional relationship to how and why you eat can actually change the way your body metabolizes food, to the point at which it can make a significant difference to your weight.

To illustrate this point, here are two startling stories, two accounts of what became, in effect, accidental but reliable scientific experiments.

The first incident took place during a study performed at Ohio State University under the direction of two scientists, Ronald Glaser and Janice Kiecollt-Glaser. These researchers wanted to show that when rabbits were fed a particular diet they would develop high cholesterol.

Their experiment did seem to prove their hypothesis, but only for about half of the rabbits. The other half of the rabbits maintained healthy levels of blood fats even though they were fed exactly the same diet as the other rabbits in the study.

The scientists were baffled, but the solution to the mystery proved to be surprisingly simple. The lab assistant who fed the rabbits would always pet and cuddle the bunnies in the lower cages but could not reach the rabbits in the upper cages. So the upper rabbits got food with no love, and their cholesterol count went up. The lower rabbits got food plus love, and their cholesterol remained healthy.

Again, both rabbits were fed the exact same diet. The only difference between the two groups was love.

The second "experiment" took place in Germany after World War II. Two state-run orphanages were run in an identical fashion: The children in each institution were given the same diet, the same doctors' visits, the same physical treatment in every way. However, one orphanage was run by a cold, critical woman who avoided contact with the children except to point out their shortcomings, frequently in public. The second orphanage was run by a warm, loving woman who comforted the children when they cried, played with them frequently, and generally expressed her caring and concern.

Despite the fact that both groups of children were given the same *physical* treatment, the ones who were given better *emotional* treatment thrived. They grew faster and gained weight, which, in this case, was a *good* thing! Love alone, it seemed, had enabled their bodies to put on extra pounds and grow taller by several inches.

In case you are wondering whether this was just a coincidence or perhaps the result of other preexisting differences between the two groups, there is scientific proof that the matrons' treatment was the key factor. As it happened, the cold, critical matron left her orphanage and the warm, loving woman was sent to replace her. As soon as the loving matron arrived, the orphans who had been struggling began to grow taller and gain much-needed weight, while the orphans who no longer had the loving matron to take care of them began to grow at a much slower rate. Loving treatment was the only variable in this experiment.

Numerous animal studies have confirmed that when animals receive loving care, they thrive. Studies of burn patients, alcoholics, nursing home residents, premature babies, and people with tuberculosis, arthritis, and heart disease further confirm these results. The power of love is an extraordinary force for health.

I will explore the impact of stress on your weight in Chapter 7, and in Chapter 8 I'll give you several specific suggestions for how to transform your experience of eating from stressful and unsatisfying into a relaxed, pleasurable, and loving experience. Here, I just want to remind you that *food is far more than a collection of chemicals and nutrients; every bite involves you in a relationship with the vegetables, fruits, and animals you consume and with the food, air, water, and soil that nourished them.*

In order to digest and metabolize your food, hundreds of intricate processes must come together within your body—hormones, enzymes, muscles, acids—along with the collective acts of trillions of tiny creatures that are not even human and yet are working together for your benefit. True nourishment comes from this set of dynamic interactions along with the dynamic interactions among farmers, animals, plants, soil, water, air, highways, truckers, grocers, clerks, refrigerator companies, power stations, and so on.

As the microbiome demonstrates, we are never just "ourselves." We are always more than ourselves—trillions of creatures more! Becoming aware of these dynamic interactions and approaching them in the spirit of love, gratitude, and appreciation can have a dynamic impact on your metabolism, weight, and health. So while you are reinoculating yourself with prebiotics and probiotics, remember also to reinoculate yourself with these powerful connections.

six

REPAIR

THE FOUR Rs
▷   **Remove**
▷   **Replace**
▷   **Reinoculate**
▼   **Repair the gut wall and the intestinal lining** by eating foods and taking supplements that support gut healt

- ▸ **Reduce inflammation with** *butyrate*, *quercitin*, and herbs like *curcumin*, which can be found in the Microbiome Super-spice *turmeric*.
- ▸ **Restore gut integrity** with the amino acid *glutamine* and with healing minerals like *zinc* among many others.
- ▸ **Replenish the crucial lining of the intestinal walls** with foods that are rich in *inulin*, *arabinogalactans*, and *fructool-igosaccharides (FOS)*:

Asparagus	Leeks
Carrots	Onion
Garlic	Radishes
Jerusalem artichoke	Tomatoes
Jicama	

continues

continued

THE FOUR RS

Reestablish intestinal balance with the correct ratio of Omega 3 to Omega 6 healthy fats:

▸ Nuts and nut butters: almond, macadamia, cashew
▸ Seeds and seed butters: sunflower seed butter
▸ Flaxseed and flaxseed oil
▸ Sunflower seed oil
▸ Olive oil

S HOSHANA WAS A FORTY-YEAR-OLD HAPPILY MARRIED MOTHER OF TWO and a dedicated high school teacher. When she first came to see me she was about twenty pounds overweight, but as we spoke I could see that was the least of her worries.

Shoshana described a multitude of symptoms that had begun to accumulate over the past several months. She was afflicted with persistent headaches, gas and bloating, severe menstrual cramps and heavy periods, frequent insomnia, and near-constant brain fog, which made her feel fuzzy, unfocused, "and just not able to get my thoughts together."

"It's like my body is just completely out of control," she told me. "I don't understand it, but I hope you can help me, Dr. Kellman, because nobody else has been able to so far."

I suspected Shoshana's extra twenty pounds, which she had gained at the same time she had acquired these painful symptoms, sprang from the same root cause that was generating all of her other problems. And after her test results came back I was even more certain.

"Shoshana," I told her, "all of your problems are related. They are all symptoms set off by an overreactive immune system, which is being triggered over and over again by a problem known as leaky gut."

I explained to Shoshana the pattern we have already discussed: An imbalanced microbiome contributed to weaknesses in her intestinal walls. Partially digested food began to leak through, setting off an immune system reaction. Soon Shoshana's immune system had made antibodies to some of these foods, and this meant she had an immune system reaction every time she ate them. Inflammation spread throughout her system, cuing her body to gain weight and disrupting her hormones, digestion, and nervous system as well as her immune system. All of her symptoms, including her weight gain, were the result of these leaky intestinal walls.

To solve Shoshana's problems we would need to restore her intestinal health and repair her gut walls along with restoring her intestinal balance. Because Shoshana had not mentioned her weight, I decided not to mention it either. Instead, I suggested she go on the Microbiome Diet as the most effective way to rebalance her microbiome, restore intestinal health, repair her gut wall, and eliminate her symptoms.

Sure enough, by the time she had completed Phase 1, most of Shoshana's symptoms had either diminished or disappeared. And, to her surprise and delight, she had also lost several pounds.

"I wasn't even trying to lose weight!" she told me. "I wasn't even *planning* to try. I just figured gaining weight is something that happens naturally as you get older."

Indeed, if you do not take care of your microbiome, you are more likely to gain weight with every passing year, but that is not because of the aging process per se; rather, it is because the assaults on your health tend to accumulate. An unhealthy diet, environmental toxins, life stress, and perhaps one or more treatments with antibiotics combine to destroy your healthy bacteria while supporting your unhealthy bacteria. Eventually your microbiome goes so far out of balance that it begins to spark inflammation, which then creates other problems. In the vicious circles we have come to know so well, an unbalanced microbiome and an inflamed system ultimately create a whole slew of problems, including weight gain, all of which are likely to keep getting worse. (For a list of symptoms of leaky gut, see the box on page 37, which lists the symptoms of an imbalanced microbiome. Because an imbalanced microbiome and leaky gut usually go together, the list of symptoms is the same.)

This process is by no means inevitable, however. Just because you are getting older does not mean you have to get less healthy. If you support your microbiome, you can maintain energy, clear thinking, good spirits, and a healthy weight no matter how old you get.

Shoshana discovered this truth by following the Microbiome Diet and seeing her symptoms disappear along with her unwanted weight. Restoring intestinal health and repairing her gut wall enabled Shoshana to regain the good health and healthy weight she had enjoyed throughout her youth. As an extra bonus, reducing her inflammation and repairing her gut gave Shoshana glowing skin, shiny hair, and a general aura of good health. When your microbiome is in balance and your digestive system is in good shape, your whole appearance shows it!

REPAIR YOUR INTESTINAL INTEGRITY

There are two portions of your digestive system you need to repair: the *microvilli* and the *tight junctions*. These are both part of the *epithelium*, the lining of the small intestine.

The tight junctions, as we have already seen, are crucial to preventing leaky gut. The tight junctions are what keep the epithelial cells close enough together so only microscopic nutrients can pass through. If the tight junctions loosen, larger portions of partially digested food can leak through, creating leaky gut and all its attendant problems.

The microvilli are long, thin projections growing out of the mucosal walls of the epithelium. I think of them as beautiful trees, waving in the breeze. Their job is to capture nutrients and pull them in toward the epithelial wall so they can be absorbed.

In a healthy gut the microvilli are flexible and robust. But in a suboptimal digestive system they tend to become atrophied. Restoring the microvilli is a crucial aspect of creating optimal digestive health. (For a list of all the factors that can undermine gut integrity, see the box on page 69.)

One of our major objectives in repairing the gut is to eliminate immune reactions to otherwise healthy foods, particularly eggs and dairy.

WHAT ABOUT TESTING?

Some practitioners recommend testing for food sensitivities, either via a blood test or through the so-called elimination test, in which you pull foods from your diet for three or more weeks and then slowly reintroduce those foods, one at a time, to see which ones you can tolerate. Usually, in an elimination test, if you are still sensitive to a food, you will have an even more extreme reaction once you reintroduce it.

I personally am not a huge fan of either the blood test or the elimination test. In my experience food sensitivities can change rapidly in both directions: You can quickly develop a sensitivity to a food you once were able to tolerate, and you can quickly develop tolerance for a food you once reacted to. I advocate focusing on the source of the problem—leaky gut. If you stay away from potentially problem foods for three weeks while healing leaky gut, you will likely be able to add many foods back. This is the protocol I follow with my patients, and it is the one I have used in the Microbiome Diet.

However, if you think you have a severe allergy with symptoms that might be disabling or life threatening, you need to go to a physician and get a different type of test known as an IGE allergy test.

In some cases, when we develop food sensitivities at a very early age or have them for many years, it becomes almost impossible to retrain the immune system. But often, once you heal the gut wall, you can indeed keep these problem foods from igniting the immune system.

REPAIR YOUR GUT WITH HEALING MINERALS AND HERBS

On the Microbiome Diet you will be using healing minerals and herbs to support your epithelial wall, restore the health of your villi, and close your tight junctions. Here is a brief look at some of the elements that will help you repair your gut.

Zinc carnosine is a combination of the mineral zinc plus the compound known as carnosine, which is composed of two amino acids, beta-alanine and l-histamine. Zinc carnosine has been shown to promote gastrointestinal healing as well as offer numerous protective benefits to the brain. Both people who have leaky gut and those with irritable bowel syndrome have been shown to be deficient in zinc as are those who suffer from obesity.

Marshmallow is not just the name of a candy; it's also the name of an herb. The plant's roots and leaves contain *mucilage*, a gluey substance that, when mixed with water, makes a slick gel that can reduce irritation by coating the throat and skin to soothe irritated mucous membranes. Marshmallow also seems to be able to coat and soothe the mucosal lining of the gut wall.

In addition, marshmallow has anti-inflammatory properties. It has been used to treat a number of conditions, including indigestion, stomach ulcers, and inflammatory bowel diseases such as Crohn's disease and ulcerative colitis.

REPAIR THE EFFECTS OF INFLAMMATION

If you have been suffering from inflammation for several years—which most dieters have—then you want to take some additional herbs and supplements to reduce your inflammation as quickly as possible. This will both improve your health and help you achieve and maintain a healthy weight.

Glutamine is a key amino acid that helps repair the intestinal wall. It provides fuel for the cells in the gastrointestinal tract and helps the whole digestive system regenerate.

Curcumin is a powerful anti-inflammatory substance found in the spice turmeric. It is also useful in treating gastrointestinal disorders and diabetes as well as reducing cholesterol.

REPAIR WITH BUTYRATE

Butyrate, or *butyric acid*, is a vital component of gut health. As we have seen, butyrate is one of the most useful short-chain fatty acids (SCFAs).

It protects against cancer, promotes immune function, heals inflammation, and improves the strength of the gut wall.

Butyrate also has significant weight loss benefits and is an integral part of our intestinal system, the primary source of energy for our large intestine. Butyrate also has anticancer and anti-inflammatory properties. As we've seen, taking prebiotics encourages your microbiome to produce short-chain fatty acids, including butyrate, but I recommend taking butyrate supplements as well.

One of my patients, Sarah, offers a dramatic example of how butyrate can affect weight. When she came to me in her early forties she had tried just about every "cutting-edge" supplement on the market: green coffee-bean extract, raspberry ketones, garcinia cambogia. Each had helped a little, but none had really made the crucial difference she needed to lose the thirty extra pounds that, she told me, "are *literally* weighing me down!"

A former dancer, Sarah felt the burden of her extra weight keenly, especially as she also had developed a runaway appetite. "Either I starve myself and suffer, or I give in and gain weight," she told me. By the time I met her she was really almost desperate to find a weight loss solution.

I loaded her up with healing foods and supplements, and I also gave her butyrate supplements. A blood test had shown me that Sarah suffered from mitochondrial dysfunction, a misfiring of the mitochondria, which produce energy within each cell. Butyrate, a few other targeted supplements, and the Microbiome Diet gave her the metabolic boost she needed. She soon began losing weight, and, she told me, she lost her outsized appetite at the same time.

To me Sarah's story exemplifies the core principle of the Microbiome Diet: Tap into the body and the microbiome's own healing wisdom, and then let nature do its magic. Why intervene and impose human control on a process that has been evolving with its own logic for millions of years? Better to work with the microbiome and the body, and let the healing begin.

REPAIR INTESTINAL BALANCE WITH HEALTHY FATS

One of the best ways to reduce inflammation is with Omega 3s, particularly in the form of EPA/DHA fish oil. In animal studies fish oil has been shown not only to reduce gut inflammation but also to help repair mucosal tissues of the digestive system. The mucosal cells of the gut wall regenerate very quickly—in a twenty-four-hour cycle—so they are very susceptible to damage. They need continual nutrition to support the cells' rapid proliferation. Fish oil supplements are an efficient way to nourish cell walls.

Vitamin B5, also known as pantothenic acid, also seems to be concentrated in gut mucosa. It too might be important for stimulating gut mucosa regeneration.

REPAIR YOUR RELATIONSHIP TO YOUR HUNGER

Hunger is a powerful word, and it's no wonder that we use "hunger" as a metaphor for many different types of desires. We hunger for food, of course, but also for love, meaning, success, quiet time, family, nature, and a better world in which to raise our children. Most of us are all too familiar with how different types of hunger can become confused, how we sometimes reach for food when we feel starved for companionship or love or how we hunger for professional success when what we really desire is meaning.

As I see it, we each contain a multitude of different worlds within us: physical, mental, emotional, spiritual. Each of these worlds leads us to hunger for what we don't yet have, and each of these hungers can be satisfied in a different way.

I believe the hunger for meaning is one of the most profound and, in our busy world, one of the least recognized. The hunger for food, by contrast, is one with which we all must contend, if only because our bodies require us to eat several times a day!

The challenge, I believe, is not to overvalue one world at the expense of the others; this book is primarily concerned with helping you repair your relationship to the physical world. But if you are feeling frustrated with issues of health and weight, you might find answers in some of the nonphysical worlds as well.

One of the best ways to repair your relationship to *any* world is to remove any impediment that short-circuits the flow of giving and receiving. If you are frustrated with your health or your weight, look at all the different worlds in which you operate: home, work, friendship, love, community, spirituality. Is there a world in which you feel unfulfilled hunger? Is there a way you might act to satisfy that hunger?

So at the same time that you are repairing your gut, you can repair your relationship to the other worlds you inhabit. Ironically, repairing these relationships can be the route to satisfying your physical hunger and to an even greater enjoyment of food.

PART III

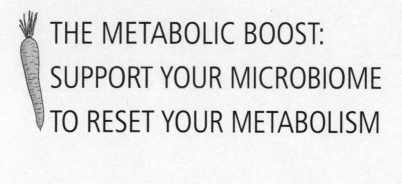

THE METABOLIC BOOST:
SUPPORT YOUR MICROBIOME
TO RESET YOUR METABOLISM

seven

STRESS CAN MAKE YOU FAT

J ACQUELINE IS A WOMAN IN HER LATE FORTIES WHO HAS ALWAYS maintained a healthy diet and a rigorous workout schedule. An energetic IT specialist, she thrives on last-minute emergencies from her roster of high-powered clients and genuinely enjoys her work. She has a loving partner with whom she has lived for the past five years, and recently the couple decided to get married. Since she was in college Jacqueline had stayed within five pounds of her ideal, healthy weight.

Then Jacqueline's widowed mother, who lived in a suburb about two hours away from Jacqueline, began to develop a mysterious condition that turned out to be a hard-to-diagnose form of dementia. Jacqueline's relationship with her mother had always been stormy, but she loved and admired her and found it very painful to witness her decline. It was also challenging to figure out where Jacqueline's mother should live and how she should be cared for, especially as the older woman insisted she was fine living on her own and became enraged at even the smallest suggestion that she might now need help.

Jacqueline came to see me because she had suddenly, mysteriously, begun to gain weight. "I'm not eating any differently than I ever have," she told me, "and because of all the stress around Mom, I'm actually exercising *more*, trying to blow off steam! This just makes no sense to me, Doctor. My last doctor told me that 'This is all just part of getting older.' I don't want to accept that—but do I have to?"

Leah, a woman in her early twenties, had moved to New York City right after graduating college and was thrilled to quickly find her niche. She loved the excitement of city life, enjoyed the circle of college friends who had also moved to New York, and told me her relationship with her boyfriend, whom she'd been dating since college, was "in a good place."

Leah had had her ups and downs with weight. In high school, she told me, she had always been a little overweight, struggling to resist the lure of French fries and desserts when she went out with her friends. Then, in college, she said, "I put on that famous Freshman Fifteen, only in my case, it was more like *twenty-five* extra pounds!" The additional weight frustrated Leah so much that, in her words, "I gave up sugar completely, stopped eating bread, and never even *looked* at a potato!"

These restrictions seemed to work for Leah, who had reached her ideal healthy weight by sophomore year and was able to maintain it all through college and into her first two years in New York.

Then Leah got a promotion. She was excited about the extra money and the new responsibilities, but she also found herself working much longer hours, responsible for many more deadlines, and in charge of managing a support staff who, as she put it, "was not always so great at getting their work done—*or* at being nice to me when I tried to get them to measure up." Although Leah insisted she had stuck to the diet that had been working for the past five years, her weight was slowly but surely creeping up, and in the past two months she had gained ten pounds.

"I'm worried it's going to *keep* getting worse, and I won't know how to stop it!" she told me. "But I haven't changed *anything*—in fact, last month I also cut out pasta! But I not only didn't lose back the old weight, I even put on a couple more pounds! What am I doing wrong?"

Michelle, a thirty-six-year-old mother of two, worked afternoons as a part-time bookkeeper. She came to see me because she had been gaining weight slowly and steadily ever since she gave birth to her first child.

"I don't understand it," she told me. "I'm really not eating any differently from before I got pregnant. I did slack off on the exercise when the kids were little, but my husband bought me an exercise bike, and now that the youngest is in nursery school I even have time to go to the gym. No matter what I do, though, the weight keeps creeping up and up and up. I'm thirty pounds heavier than I was five years ago. Am I doomed to gain another thirty pounds in the next five years?"

Will, an energetic, ambitious man in his midforties, prided himself on being only ten pounds heavier than he was in college without ever putting much effort into diet or exercise. Will enjoyed his job as an IT specialist at a large Manhattan company, was happy in his marriage to his college sweetheart, and was proud of his two healthy, thriving teenage children.

Then his younger son, Liam, left middle school for high school, and suddenly the problems began. Liam's grades fell off. He no longer spent time with his old friends and seemed to have difficulty making new ones. He looked for any excuse to avoid spending time with his family. Will and his wife were at a loss.

After a month or so Will began to notice that he himself was putting on weight, slowly but surely. He cut out desserts, started working out on his wife's treadmill, and even gave up the beers he used to enjoy while watching football on Sunday afternoons. Despite these efforts the new pounds didn't go away, and in fact, Will's weight continued to rise. He came to me anxious both about his son and about himself.

Jacqueline, Leah, Michelle, and Will were all experiencing a very common phenomenon: Stress was causing them to gain or retain weight. Scientists have long known that stress is a major cause of weight gain, including physical stressors like insufficient sleep and missed meals, as well as psychological stressors, such as a sick family member, pressing deadlines, challenging relationships, or the intense demands of parenting. Now that we know more about the microbiome, we understand that stress also affects our inner ecology in ways that both threaten our health and increase our weight.

Stress promotes weight gain in a number of ways:

- **Excess stress produces imbalances in *cortisol*,** a stress hormone that, at the right levels, makes you feel energized and alive but at the wrong levels encourages your body to hold onto every last bit of fat, no matter how little you eat or how much you exercise.
- **Excess stress compromises gut integrity** and contributes to leaky gut. And, as we have seen, leaky gut creates inflammation, a major factor in obesity, weight gain, and fat retention.
- **Stress alters the composition of the microbiome.** As we have also seen, an imbalanced microbiome contributes to inflammation, leaky gut, and digestive difficulties, all of which further stress your body.

All of these stress-related factors cue your body to store fat rather than burn it. Together they create a vicious cycle that can make it seemingly impossible to lose unwanted weight.

YOUR FAT IS NOT YOUR FAULT, PART 2

I often tell my patients who are facing stressful situations that their fat is not their fault. I'll tell you the same thing and for the same reason: *your biology is cued to hold onto weight whenever it perceives you to be under stress.*

This makes sense when you consider that the gravest danger our early ancestors faced was lack of food. In a subsistence world you needed body fat to protect you against the cold as well as to tide you

How Stress Undermines Your Digestive System and Your Weight

- Changes the chemicals your stomach secretes, interfering with digestion
- Decreases hydrochloric acid (stomach acid), also interfering with digestion
- Keeps your food from moving smoothly through your gut
- Promotes leaky gut
- Changes blood flow to the mucous membranes that line your gut walls and absorb nutrients
- Alters your microbiome, leading to inflammation, insulin resistance, and weight gain
- Promotes fat storage in the abdomen, where it creates the greatest health risks
- Affects your blood sugar metabolism, causing you to crave more fatty and sugary foods
- Increases the cortisol, a stress hormone, in your system, which promotes insulin resistance and fat storage
- Lowers testosterone and decreases muscle mass, which slows down your metabolism

over when food was scarce. Our bodies evolved to respond to any type of stress—physical or emotional—by holding onto fat, literally for dear life.

Now I'm not giving you this information to stress you further! As you can see from the examples of Jacqueline, Leah, Michelle, and Will, many types of stress are unavoidable or even welcome. Jacqueline chose to care for her elderly mother, Leah was delighted about her promotion, and both Michelle and Will generally enjoyed being parents. None of these people really had the option of simply avoiding the stressful situations in which they found themselves.

But this does not mean they—or you—are doomed to remain overweight. The goal is not to strive for an unrealistic fantasy of a stress-free life but rather to figure out what kind of support your body needs to feel "safe" rather than "stressed."

So here's the good news: *supporting your body during challenging times can counteract the stress response and reboot your metabolism to burn fat instead of store it.*

The Microbiome Diet provides you with the physical support you need to counter the effects of stress. If you follow the Microbiome Diet—even with the 70 percent compliance you can maintain in Phase 3—you will be getting all the nutrients you need to support your microbiome, your digestive system, and your brain. This in turn will help balance your production of stress hormones, leaving you with stress chemicals at just the right levels to feel energized and motivated rather than at the levels that cue your body to retain weight.

Stress-free eating, which I'll explain to you in Chapter 8, will also go a long way toward recuing your stress response, supporting your digestive system, and restoring a healthy microbiome.

So let's look at all the ways stress can make you fat. I believe that when you understand how stress leads to weight gain, you will feel liberated from the frustration and confusion of watching your weight continue to climb. Instead, you can feel empowered, excited, and confident in your ability to achieve and maintain a healthy weight.

SOCIAL STRESS: WHEN LIFE CIRCUMSTANCES CONSPIRE TO MAKE YOU FAT

When you start to put on weight without changing your diet or exercise routine you might easily feel as though you're slowly going crazy. Perhaps you can't believe that you really *are* eating the same

---

CONSTANT DIETING CAN PACK ON THE POUNDS

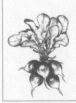

Efforts to restrict what you eat can be another type of physical and emotional stress. Some studies suggest that continual dieting produces increases in cortisol levels of as much as 18 percent. Cortisol promotes insulin resistance, which in turn promotes fat storage, especially around the abdomen.

amounts, especially because your family, friends, and physician are likely to doubt your word. You might obsessively review every bite you took, desperately searching for the "forbidden food" that somehow caused the problem. If you used to be able to indulge in an occasional dessert or high-fat food without gaining weight, you might even feel guilty, as though you had somehow been "getting away" with something that now has caught up to you.

But what if you could see exactly how powerful stress can be when it comes to weight gain?

Looking at studies conducted with animals really drives home the point that *stress creates fat storage*. After all, animals don't eat because they are lonely or scared! Their psychology and willpower are not the issue—the only factor is their biology. So if stressed animals overeat, eat in an unhealthy pattern, or gain weight even when their calories are restricted, we can see with crystal clarity that stress and weight gain are a matter of biology.

And in fact, numerous experiments show that animals put into stressful situations gain weight, even when they are eating exactly the same food as before, even when they are eating exactly the same food as the unstressed animals who do *not* gain weight.

So many studies have been done on stress and weight that in 2012 a team of researchers at the University of Cincinnati College of Medicine decided to get an overview, reviewing both human and animal studies on the relationship of stress and obesity. The Cincinnati researchers concluded that, indeed, a great deal of evidence suggests a link between chronic stress and belly fat. They also found that stress tends to change the way you eat, leading you to crave "nutrient-dense 'comfort foods.'"

Of course, most of us are familiar with the idea that if you are unhappy, anxious, or stressed, you tend to seek comfort foods that are likely to be high in starches, sugars, and fats. Significantly, the Cincinnati researchers showed this is a pattern among animals as well as humans, suggesting there is a biological link, not just a psychological one, between chronic stress and the craving for foods that are more likely to lead to fat storage.

These findings make sense if we recall that for most humans and animals in the wild stress indicates a physically challenging situation. Maybe you have to run from a predator, exert yourself to search for scarce food, or migrate from one home to another. Perhaps the stress you face *is* a lack of food, and your anxiety is because the dominant animals in the group will get more of whatever food there is, leaving you in danger of starvation.

This is still the situation for animals in the wild, and it was certainly the case for humans throughout most of our time on this planet. And so when your body feels endangered you eat as much as you can get when you can get it, you crave the foods that will turn into fat, and you adjust your metabolism to hold onto that fat. All of those are protective devices in a situation in which you can't be sure of having ready access to food—although they obviously are not so useful in helping you cope with a sick mother, a stressful job, or the challenges of parenting!

By contrast, when your body feels safe you are more likely to burn fat rather than store it. Your body interprets "less stress" as "more confident about getting food" and "less likely to face physical challenges that require stored body fat." So feeling less stress cues your body to burn fat rather than store it.

Eating patterns are a significant part of weight gain, so it's significant that they, too, have been correlated with stress. A 2010 study by a different team of University of Cincinnati researchers, led by Susan J. Melhorn, found that weight gain was correlated with social stress and with long-term metabolic changes that might lead to obesity. This experiment also looked at eating patterns, exploring why some rats in the study chose to eat frequent, small meals while others chose to eat fewer and bigger meals.

Eating patterns are important, because we've known for a while that eating fewer and larger meals promotes weight gain and body fat retention as well as increasing triglycerides and cholesterol. In fact, if you eat three large meals each day, you are more likely to boost triglycerides and cholesterol than if you eat five smaller meals, even if you consume the same number of calories. Likewise, you are less likely to gain weight when you choose smaller, more frequent meals, even if you overeat.

The Melhorn team wanted to find out whether there was any relationship between stress and eating patterns. So they began with a group of rats that were formed into colonies, which quickly produced a hierarchy of one dominant male and three subordinates.

While the rats were forming the hierarchy they all ate less—and lost weight. But once the hierarchy was formed, the dominant rats ate more, while the subordinate rats ate less.

This makes sense. Access to food is the most important benefit an animal or human can enjoy, so we might expect the dominant animals to use their power to gain greater access to food. Significantly, though, the dominant rats ate smaller and more frequent meals. The subordinate animals ate less often, but they made up for it by consuming bigger meals when they did eat. Perhaps, having less control over when they got access to food, the subordinate animals wanted to take advantage of whatever access they did get by eating as much as possible and storing up body fat just in case they had to wait a while before they ate again.

After two weeks the colonies were broken up and the male rats were housed individually for three weeks. During that period they were allowed to eat freely, with no other rats to compete for their supply of food.

Both the dominant and the subordinate rats overate during their three-week access to unlimited food. But the dominant rats continued to eat more frequent and smaller meals, while the subordinate rats kept on with their pattern of less frequent and larger meals. The dominant rats did gain both weight and body mass, but the subordinate rats gained more belly fat.

What can we conclude from this?

First, stress and feeling "on the bottom" of the social scale cues your biology to choose larger and less frequent meals, perhaps because you're afraid of having less access to food. Remember, this is a pattern chosen by rats, so psychological factors, such as "comfort food," "stuffing down feelings," or any other emotions related to food, really aren't an issue. *Biologically*, feeling stressed and subordinate led the rats to eat in a way that made them more likely to gain not just weight but belly fat.

Second, the experience of being subordinate or dominant seemed to create long-lasting metabolic changes in both groups of rats. Even when they had unlimited access to food and could eat whenever they wanted, the dominant rats chose the eating pattern that helped them resist weight gain and made them less likely to acquire belly fat. Their metabolism had grown accustomed to this pattern, and they maintained it even when their circumstances had changed.

Likewise, even when the subordinate rats had the opportunity to eat freely they continued in the patterns they had developed when they were competing with the dominant rats for food. They chose an eating pattern that was biologically guaranteed to pack on the belly fat and raise their triglycerides and cholesterol. These ongoing metabolic changes basically doomed them to gain unhealthy weight.

Fortunately, unlike rats, we can choose to alter our eating patterns, support our microbiome, and transform our relationship to food. Even if, like Jacqueline, Leah, Michelle, and Will, you cannot quickly change the circumstances stressing you out, you *can* change your relationship to those circumstances. More important, you can change the attitude you bring to the table and the degree of stress you invite to every meal. In Chapter 8 I'll show you how to change that vital relationship so that you too can cue your metabolism to burn fat and bring you to a healthy weight.

STRESS, FAT, AND YOUR MICROBIOME

A healthy microbiome is crucial to maintaining a healthy weight. However, stress rapidly destroys many of the healthy bacteria we need. In fact, the microbiome is so sensitive that even twenty-four hours' worth of stress can significantly change its population.

This makes sense when you consider that the microbes in our microbiome have a life span of about twenty minutes. So a twenty-four-hour day is seventy-two lifetimes to them, the equivalent of fifteen hundred years in human time!

Over those fifteen hundred "microbe years" healthy bacteria die and unhealthy bacteria move in to take their place. As a result, you can go from a fat-burning system to a fat-storing system in the span of just one stressful day, especially if you are not eating the foods and taking the probiotics to keep your microbiome in balance.

Every time you unbalance your microbiome you weaken your digestive system, set yourself up for leaky gut, and become more likely to gain belly fat. So when you think about the effects of stress, picture the following chain of events:

stress ➡ unbalanced microbiome ➡ disrupted metabolism ➡ weight gain

In one fascinating study conducted in 2011 a group of researchers had mice share a cage with more aggressive mice—one clever way scientists have of stressing mice! The mice forced to deal with the aggressors suffered a loss in beneficial bacteria, less overall diversity in their gut microbiome, and an increase in harmful bacteria, making them more vulnerable to infection and creating intestinal inflammation, all leading straight to weight gain.

Most of us would agree that exam week is a stressful time for university students. So we might expect that students' microbiomes would undergo a change between the relatively relaxed first few days of school to the stressful time of final exams. And indeed, in 2008 an Australian team of researchers conducted a study that found exactly that: students had fewer healthy bacteria during exam week than they had had at the beginning of the semester.

But here's what turns the whole process into a truly vicious cycle: An unhealthy microbiome isn't just the effect of stress—it can also be the *cause* of stress. Studies have shown that an imbalanced microbiome can lead to greater anxiety and depression. When your microbiome is out of balance you just don't feel right. And your body can interpret this "not rightness" as a danger that causes it to hold onto fat.

YOUR BRAIN AND YOUR 'BIOME

Remember how I explained in Part I that the gut is actually a second brain? After all, it produces many of the neurotransmitters that your brain needs, the biochemicals through which your brain regulates thought and emotion.

Well, the microbiome is like the command center of that second brain. And its power to affect our thoughts and feelings is truly remarkable.

The trillions of bacteria living inside you can cause you to crave sugar, starches, and greasy foods. They can keep you from thinking clearly, disrupt your concentration, and interfere with your memory. They can affect how intensely you feel pain and how quickly you respond to stress. They can even cause you to feel anxious and depressed. Whenever my patients tell me they "just can't think right," "can't remember a darn thing," or "feel like my brain is broken," the first thing I check out is their microbial balance and digestive health.

Why do the bacteria inside you have such power? Because they have a tremendous impact on the biochemicals that your brain uses to process thought and emotion. Your nervous system, your hormones, and your immune system are all involved in the complicated chemical signaling that goes on between your brain, your gut, and your microbiome.

Specifically, your microbiome is crucial in determining whether your gut is able to produce the right chemicals in the right amounts. Accordingly, imbalance in the microbiome disrupts the gut, which in turn can produce such symptoms as brain fog, memory issues, anxiety, and depression:

imbalanced microbiome

⬇

disrupted gastrointestinal system

⬇

incorrect levels of neurotransmitters (brain chemicals)

⬇

symptoms of poor thinking and altered mood

Conversely, when your microbiome is in balance and your gut is functioning at optimal levels your biochemicals are likely to be in balance. You feel calm, clear, focused, energized, and optimistic. When a challenge arises you are confident you can meet it. When you encounter a problem, you feel motivated to confront it and are able to bear down on the problem and stick with it until it is solved. When a stressful situation makes demands on your physical, mental, or emotional energy, you are able to keep things in perspective, remain positive, and summon the stamina to soldier on.

balanced microbiome
⬇
healthy gastrointestinal system
⬇
correct levels of neurotransmitters (brain chemicals)
⬇
clear thinking and calm, confident, energetic mood

When you have to face a stressful situation you want your microbiome to be balanced and healthy, both for your emotional well-being and to keep from gaining weight. After all, 90 percent of our body's serotonin, the chemical that enables us to feel calm, optimistic, and self-confident, is manufactured in the gut, and the health of your microbiome affects your serotonin levels. We also know that gut bacteria both produce and respond to other chemicals that the brain uses to create thoughts and feelings, including melatonin, which regulates sleep; the "stress chemicals" dopamine and norepinephrine; and the "relaxation chemicals" acetylcholine and GABA.

INFLAMMATION AND YOUR BRAIN

Another factor that can disrupt brain chemistry is inflammation, which results both from leaky gut and from an imbalanced microbiome. People with high levels of inflammation may be more susceptible to anxiety and depression. In fact, more than half of people suffering from such chronic gastrointestinal disorders as ulcerative colitis, Crohn's disease, and irritable bowel syndrome (IBS) also show symptoms of stress, anxiety, and depression. IBS has also been associated with increased reactions to pain.

Researchers studying the brain-gut-microbiome axis are confident that further research will reveal still more ways in which the microbiome influences our feelings, thoughts, and behavior.

THE POWER OF PROBIOTICS

If the microbiome has such an enormous impact on our memory, thought, and mood, it follows that taking probiotics would have a demonstrable effect on memory, stress, and other mental/emotional functions.

A 2010 experiment involved a Canadian team of researchers who disrupted the microbiome of a group of mice by infecting them with a specific type of harmless bacteria. When these mice were exposed to acute stress, they had memory problems within about ten days. However, those problems were prevented by giving the mice a daily dose of probiotics, which presumably helped their microbiomes restore a healthy balance. Other studies on both animals and humans have also shown that probiotics reduce anxiety and soothe the stress response as well as boost mood in patients with IBS and chronic fatigue syndrome. A 2011 experiment discovered that thirty days' worth of treatment with probiotics led healthy humans to feel less anxiety and depression.

We don't yet know all the answers as to why probiotics combat depression, but scientists speculate that probiotics decrease inflammation and support the production of *tryptophan*, a neurotransmitter that is a precursor to *serotonin*. Serotonin is the ultimate feel-good brain chemical, making us feel calm, balanced, optimistic, and self-confident. Higher levels of serotonin help us combat depression. And of course, because 90 percent of our serotonin is made in the gut, probiotics probably support the microbiome in its efforts to maintain gut health.

In 2013 a study from UCLA provided further evidence that probiotics improve brain function, particularly with regard to depression, anxiety, and stress. In this groundbreaking study thirty-six women aged eighteen to fifty-five were divided into three groups. One group ate a yogurt that contained a mix of several probiotics. They consumed this microbiome-friendly food twice a day for four weeks.

probiotics ➡ balanced microbiome ➡ healthier gut walls ➡ more serotonin ➡ less depression/anxiety

A second group ate a dairy product that looked and tasted like the yogurt but contained no probiotics. The third group was not given anything special to eat in the experiment.

Then the women were given FMRI scans with their brains at rest and during an emotion-recognition task in which they viewed a series of pictures of people with angry or frightened faces and had to match those images to pictures of other people showing those emotions.

The women who had been given probiotics were less stressed during the test and showed more connections between various regions of the brain. Likewise, in another recent study people who were given probiotics reported less anxiety, depression, and anger as well as an improved ability to solve problems.

So it seems the microbiome mediates the stress response as well as other brain functions. A healthy microbiome enables you to react to challenging situations with less stress and more ease. This is significant for mood, mental function, and weight loss, because, as we have seen, stress promotes fat storage. So this is yet another way in which a healthy microbiome enables you to achieve a healthy weight:

healthy microbiome ➡ healthier stress response ➡ fewer stress chemicals ➡ fewer fat-storing cues

THE EMPOWERING DIET

The relationship between stress and weight is complex because there are two different types of stress response. One type is known as "fight or flight," the way the body mobilizes itself to make extraordinary efforts in pursuit of a goal. The nickname comes from imagining our ancestors, who had to fight enemies or flee predators, but as we have seen, this type of stress response can also involve sustained, prolonged effort—pulling a capsized fishing boat out of the surf, for example, or trekking across the tundra to a new home.

In the "fight or flight" type of stress, hormones such as cortisol, adrenaline, and dopamine serve as a way to mobilize our resources. This response sends added strength to our muscles and causes us to breathe more deeply so we can support a more rapid heartbeat and increased blood flow. I think of the "fight or flight" stress response as optimistic, as we hope to outrun our predators, defeat our enemies, or complete the demanding efforts needed to improve our lives.

But there is another, more deadly response to prolonged, chronic stress: the *defeat response*. When we are subjected to ongoing and seemingly endless stress, sometimes our will to fight or flee breaks down. Rather than mobilizing our bodies and emotions for extraordinary effort, we brace ourselves to face the crushing blows we believe will inevitably come.

Whether it's a difficult job full of frustrating, meaningless tasks and abusive treatment from your boss or that your relationship, friendships, and social life are not really fulfilling, this sense of defeat and demoralization creates another type of stress response, one with even more serious consequences for weight gain. It has been associated with retention of body fat, especially around the abdomen, along with obesity and the suppression of the immune system.

So many of the patients I see in my practice come in feeling terribly disempowered. They feel "the system"—whatever that means to them—is indifferent, impermeable, and far more powerful than they are. They feel undervalued. And they feel their true selves have been buried beneath a deep layer of defeat. They have the sense that forces far more powerful than they are—the economy, the culture, the media, job difficulties, family pressures—are taking advantage of them and that there is nothing they can do but just follow along.

These feelings are especially problematic when it comes to food. If you feel disempowered, how are you going to challenge the unhealthy food culture in which we live, where so many items are processed, packaged, and preserved; where so many items are genetically altered; where gluten, corn, sweeteners, and unhealthy fats are added to almost everything? That sense of defeat leads people simply to "follow the script," eating the foods that are convenient—easy to obtain, easy to include in your daily routine, easy to pick up at the supermarket or order at the nearest restaurant.

So many unhealthy food choices surround us, in high-end bistros as well as fast food restaurants, in upscale groceries as well as budget stores. Whether you're buying luxury items or low-priced bargains, so many food choices are loaded with unhealthy fat, extra sugar, high-fructose corn syrup, processed soy, and gluten. So many food choices are stripped of nutrients and freshness. So many choices are guaranteed to set off cravings, inflame your system, and keep you permanently hungry even as you continue to gain weight.

What enables you to navigate this overwhelming food culture with its seductive, unhealthy choices?

In my experience, to eat consistently in a healthy way you need to be in touch with your own inner power, the power that springs from knowing your true self. When you access your true self you also access your true hunger. You get a real sense of what your body needs as well as what you crave emotionally and spiritually. Your true self leads you to feed each hunger with the nourishment it truly desires. Yes, sometimes that is food. But sometimes what you really crave is some quiet time, a hug, an exciting adventure, or a deeper sense of connection to something larger than yourself.

When you have rebalanced your inner ecology your whole system finds its balance as well. You are more in touch with your body, your emotions, and your mental power. You have the opportunity to find out what truly tastes delicious to you—not the processed, packaged, ready-made choices made by the gargantuan food industry but rather your own personal tastes and delights. And you have the mental and emotional energy to pursue what is truly important to you.

eight

STRESS-FREE EATING CAN HELP YOU LOSE WEIGHT

JOHNETTA WAS AN EXUBERANT WOMAN IN HER LATE FORTIES WHO TOLD me on our first visit that she had always been big: "big voice, big personality, and a plus-sized woman!" She was concerned about her weight, though, because of a family history of diabetes on her father's side and heart disease on her mother's side.

When Johnetta learned the principles of the Microbiome Diet and about the foods she would be focused on during the first two weeks of Phase 1, she said, "I won't lie to you, Doctor—it's going to be hard." Johnetta hated the idea of giving up the soul food diet she had enjoyed with her family growing up in Atlanta, as those were the foods she associated with family warmth, good times, and love. Macaroni and cheese, yams mashed with brown sugar, collard greens stewed with ham, and fried chicken were the cuisine of her childhood, and even though she could allow herself some of those foods in Phase 2 and Phase 3, with only 90 percent and 70 percent compliance, respectively, she still felt sad about steering the majority of her diet in such a new direction.

"Well," I said after a moment's thought, "what *else* do you associate with those family dinners?"

Johnetta looked at me and shook her head. "I don't understand."

"It wasn't only the food that made those times special," I said. "What else made your family dinners so good?"

Slowly Johnetta's face lit up. She described the laughing and joking around the dinner table, the feeling of safety and comfort she enjoyed as a child, the sense that the world was full of people who loved her and would take care of her. She also enjoyed joking and getting into mischief with her cousins when they all met for Sunday dinners, and she remembered getting advice from two of her older cousins when she was just starting to get interested in boys.

I asked Johnetta to tell me about other meals that were special to her. She described a romantic date with "the *then* love of my life," at which the two had lingered for hours over course after course of delicious food at a candlelit dinner in a Paris café. "It sounds *so* corny," she said with a sigh. "But it was *so* special." She also remembered the local bar near her first job where she and two work friends would meet on Friday afternoons to snack on appetizers and sip wine as they blew off steam about work and gave each other support about "work, love, family, and everything under the sun!"

"So," I told Johnetta, "the food is one part of the meal, but *who* you ate with, *how* you ate, and what happened *while* you ate were at least as important."

Each of the meals she had described was a form of "stress-free eating," which was fundamentally different from eating in a rush, while working, or when anxious. I also told Johnetta that whether she ate alone or in company, she could always create a stress-free environment around her food in which she felt connected to the love and pleasure in her life and enjoyed her food to the utmost. Eating in a stress-free way, I told her, was just as important a part of her weight loss as the actual food.

As we saw in Chapter 7, the connection between food and stress is demonstrated scientifically through numerous animal studies. It is a biological fact I have seen confirmed among my own patients time and time again. Stressed eating leads to weight gain. Stress-free eating helps you lose weight. It really is that simple.

There are three ways to reduce stress during mealtimes:

- Focused eating
- Invoking gratitude and appreciation
- Eating with love

Each of these might be appropriate in different situations. All of them can help you achieve and maintain a healthy weight.

FOCUSED EATING

Focused eating is also called "mindful eating," in acknowledgment of the Buddhist teachings of mindfulness. Focusing on just one thing—just the thing you are doing at the time—is part of the Buddhist principle of living, fully awake, in the present. Instead of allowing your mind to wander toward the future, which cannot truly be known, or toward the past, which cannot ever be changed, you focus completely on each moment as you live it—fully aware, fully present.

You don't have to be a Buddhist to take advantage of this insight. Just imagine for a moment how different this attitude is from the one most of us usually bring to the table, especially when we are eating alone. We distract ourselves with television or a book or we turn our thoughts to problems at work, relationship issues, or other stressful topics. We might even work while we eat, barely aware of the food we are consuming, numb to its tastes and textures and aromas, insensitive to the pleasure it might bring us. This is also the way we often drink coffee or tea—not using these flavorful beverages to create a mini-oasis of pleasure and relaxation but as the barely noticed accompaniment to meeting a deadline or trying to get through yet another meeting.

Focused eating, by contrast, invites you to fully experience all the delights of the food before you—the tangy crispness of an apple, the dill-scented richness of a meaty borscht, the earthy green taste of a spinach salad. Chewing slowly, you notice the way flavor fills your mouth. As you swallow, you experience the sensation of feeling full and satisfied. You feel the comforting warmth of the food in your stomach and the mental shift as your newly nourished brain perks up. The sensuous delights of your food and the sensual pleasure of chewing, swallowing, and digesting are so fulfilling that the entire experience of eating shifts from the stressful, distracted fashion in which we normally consume foods.

I deeply believe that once you have begun to nourish your microbiome, focused eating is perhaps your second most powerful weapon in your battle to achieve a healthy weight. Focused eating decreases stress, and this supports the microbiome.

Focused eating also lowers cortisol levels, reversing the metabolic pattern of storing belly fat. Lower cortisol creates less inflammation, and, as we have seen, inflammation cues your system to store fat instead of burn it.

Finally, focused eating causes you to eat less because every bite is so satisfying. You are feeding your senses and emotions as well as your body. Because you are getting more satisfaction in every way, you need less food.

Too often when we feel hungry we go to the refrigerator, not bothering to ask whether our hunger is for food or perhaps instead for companionship, comfort, or meaning. If you eat in a focused, mindful way, with every bite a rich, sensuous experience, you will find yourself hungry for food when you really do need to nourish your physical self and hungry for something else when another part of you is hungry. This awareness of what you are really hungry for will help you achieve your ideal weight while freeing you from feeling that your hunger and cravings are beyond your control.

INVOKING GRATITUDE AND APPRECIATION

As I think about the world my own young daughters will grow up in I can't help feeling sad that many children today have no real idea of where food comes from. For too many of our children food is something that comes packaged from a grocery store. They can't even envision that vegetables were once growing in the ground and had to be nurtured by a farmer or that fruit was once growing on a vine or a tree and had to be picked and stored and shipped so we can eat them.

Feeling grateful for the food you eat and appreciating every aspect of how it got to your table is a wonderful stress reliever and a terrific way to shift the chemical processes within your body as you encounter a meal. Remember, our goal is to lower cortisol and create a physically healthy response to tasting, chewing, swallowing, and digesting. Taking a moment before eating to focus on what you are consuming and appreciate the journey it took to your plate will nudge your chemical responses to that food into a calmer, more pleasurable place. By lowering your stress hormones, appreciation will help cue your body chemistry toward feeling full when you really have had enough and toward burning fat rather than storing it.

As we saw in Chapter 7, the stress response is a biochemical shift within your body that resembles the processes mice, rats, and monkeys undergo. When animals are stressed or feel "subordinate" they gain weight—specifically, belly fat. They also develop metabolic patterns that cue them to remain hungry, overeat, and keep gaining weight. Because this is the experience of animals, we know it is a biological response, not necessarily a psychological one.

But even though we are animals, we are not *only* animals! No one would ever ask a mouse to be grateful for its chow or expect a monkey to appreciate the work that went into growing a banana. We, however, can nurture our own feelings of gratitude and appreciation as we approach the table. In doing so, we cue our bodies to let go, at least temporarily, of the stresses and subordination in our lives, thereby altering our cortisol levels, supporting our digestion, destressing our immune system, and boosting our metabolism.

If we too were in the wild, we might be grateful for the evolutionary process that cues our body to hold onto fat whenever we feel stressed, endangered, or socially subordinate. But because we are not in the wild, we can be grateful we have the mental and emotional resources to shift those biological patterns! Feeling gratitude and appreciation for our food sounds like a mushy, sentimental idea, but I assure you it is not! It is hard science, a way to alter the cortisol response that, as we saw in Chapter 7, causes stressed animals to gain weight even while consuming the exact same food as their unstressed counterparts.

THE FRENCH PARADOX

As the obesity epidemic rises in the United States we continue to puzzle over the so-called French paradox. The typical French meal contains butter, flour, sugar, salt—rich sauces, crispy French bread, a luscious dessert, and, of course, a glass or two of wine. Yet the French, by and large, remain at healthy weights. Why?

Nutritionists and researchers have puzzled over this problem for years, and a wide variety of theories have been propounded. I am sure many of them have merit, but I know one key factor, at least, is the attitude the French bring to each meal.

The French eat slowly, chewing their food and savoring its flavors. Even when they eat in fast food restaurants, they typically take more time there than the average American. They tend to eat in company, in an atmosphere of sociability, enjoying the conversation, the connections, the closeness of family or the companionship of friends.

If you can eat with those you love and if you can find a way to make these meals an occasion for companionship and closeness, you too can benefit from at least some aspects of the "French paradox." Simply put, this is another way to shift the stress response, which exerts a strong biological pull in the direction of fat retention and weight gain. Making your meals a time to feel love and pleasure is a key resource for transforming your body chemistry and boosting your metabolism.

A GUIDED TOUR OF YOUR GASTROINTESTINAL SYSTEM

Knowing how the food makes its journey from your plate to your weight will help you focus on the sensations of eating, chewing, and digesting, thus enhancing your mindfulness and pleasure at the table. So here is a closer look at what goes on when you first reach for, say, a slice of apple.

The first thing to notice is that digestion begins in the brain. You see the piece of apple, smell its faint fragrance, feel its soft, uneven texture between your fingers. These sensory experiences begin in your brain and are enough to cue your entire digestive system to get ready to do its job. When we talk about *mouthwatering* smells, that is not simply a metaphor; it is a literal description of reality. A smell—in fact, the mere idea of food—can trigger a response from your salivary glands as they prepare your body to absorb the approaching nutrients.

I'll show you exactly what I mean. As you read this page pause for a moment to evoke the smells, tastes, and textures of your favorite food. Really bring that food to life in as much sensory detail as possible. Picture the food just before you begin to take a bite. Remember how that food tastes and smells. Feel its texture and temperature in your mouth.

If you have really brought a favorite food to mind, you might notice that your mouth waters, your stomach almost growls, and you actually begin to feel hungry. That is the power of your brain over your digestive system. As your brain envisions the prospect of food, whether real or imaginary, your mouth waters, producing salivary enzymes that will start breaking down your food as soon as it reaches your mouth. These enzymes are an important part of the digestive process, as we saw in Chapter 4, and they also help to kill any foreign bacteria that do not belong in your system.

At the same time, your digestive system also begins to produce enzymes, while your hormones, including those that create hunger and fullness, begin to flow. During times of stress your blood flows into your outer muscles—your arms and legs—so you can either fight or flee. By contrast, when your brain anticipates food your blood moves inward, helping your stomach to receive your food and your intestinal walls to pass it through. That's why it's such a bad idea to eat when you are stressed: Your blood is divided between helping you digest and helping you take action. When food enters your body you want all your resources mobilized to help you digest.

In fact, your nervous system contains two major subsystems—one to help your body act and one to help it rest. The *sympathetic* nervous system, which produces the stress response, cues your body for fight or flight. The *parasympathetic* nervous system, which produces the relaxation response, cues your body to "rest and digest."

Our bodies were never meant to digest food in "fight or flight" mode, as is made clear by the flow of blood and hormones associated with that response. Stress makes our heart race, pumps blood quickly through our bodies, and prepares us to move quickly and vigorously to cope with necessity or danger.

Relaxation, by contrast, slows our heart rate, lowers our blood pressure, and cues us to calmly absorb nutrients from the foods we swallow. The parasympathetic state is also where healing takes place. It is the "down time" that we need to recover, rejuvenate, and restore our bodies after the exertions of the stress response.

It can be hard to activate the parasympathetic nervous system, especially when we face chronic, persistent stress. This is why I recommend taking a moment before you eat and consciously trying to shift from one system to the other. The techniques described later in this chapter can help you do that.

EATING SLOW AND FEELING FULL

As soon as you take food into your mouth you begin to chew, which releases more saliva. *Amylase*, an enzyme in your saliva, helps your body prepare to digest carbohydrates—grains, vegetables, fruits, and sweets.

The more thoroughly you chew your food, the more thoroughly you prepare it for digestion. Most of us don't chew our food completely enough; it's as though, seeking instant gratification, we are trying simply to swallow it whole. But one of the best things you can do for your weight as well as your health is to slow down your meal times. And one of the best ways to slow down your meals is to chew more.

There are many ways in which chewing more thoroughly will help you lose weight. First, the hormones that signal fullness, including leptin, don't peak until between twenty to forty minutes after you have begun eating. If you wolf down your food, you basically trick your body into letting you overeat. That same stressful response also cues your body to store fat rather than burn it. Those might be good strategies for someone living in a culture where food is scarce and the next meal is uncertain, but it's a terrible idea for anyone who wants to lose weight. If you eat slowly, you are far more likely to eat no more than your body really needs, because you give your feelings of fullness a chance to kick in.

THE POWER OF POSITIVE CHEWING

Chewing itself is also a powerful stress reliever, as a number of studies have shown. Most of these studies relate to chewing gum, but the principle is the same either way.

A group of researchers at Swinburne University in Melbourne, Australia, conducted a study finding that chewing gum lowered

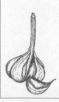

WHY STRESS-FREE EATING HELPS YOU LOSE WEIGHT	
Sympathetic Nervous System	**Parasympathetic Nervous System**
"fight or flight"	"rest and digest"
blood flows to extremities	blood flows to digestive organs
chronic stress triggers fat storage	eating while relaxed interrupts chronic stress and triggers fat burning

cortisol levels. Remember, cortisol is associated with the "fight or flight" stress response. I wonder if perhaps chewing cues the body to switch from that "fight or flight" response to the "rest and digest" response instead. Perhaps by chewing your food longer you are giving your body more time to switch from stressing to relaxing, which also helps you switch from fat storage to fat burning.

THE STOMACH'S STORY

After chewing comes swallowing, as your food makes its way down your esophagus and into your stomach. There it is greeted by hydrochloric acid and the enzyme known as pepsin.

The saliva in your mouth has already begun to break down carbs. But proteins and fats don't begin to be digested until they hit the acid in your stomach. As your stomach acid breaks apart the protein molecules, pepsin ruptures the bonds between amino acids, making the protein chains shorter and more digestible.

Hydrochloric acid also kills microbes. As saliva is your first line of defense against unfriendly bacteria, stomach acid is your second. Stomach acid is crucial in preventing the overgrowth of unhealthy bacteria and, therefore, helps keep your microbiome in balance.

When you're stressed or struggling with an unhealthy microbiome, your stomach acid levels decrease. This compromises your digestion and also allows unhealthy bacteria to start colonizing your digestive system. So here's another vicious cycle:

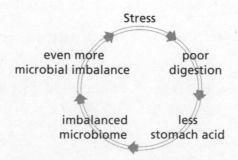

Stress

even more
microbial imbalance

poor
digestion

imbalanced
microbiome

less
stomach acid

As we saw in Chapter 4, low stomach acid can be yet another factor that stresses your system, triggers cortisol production, slows your metabolism, and cues your body to store fat rather than burn it. It can also cause acid reflux, which many physicians mistakenly treat with antacids or proton pump inhibitors. Because you don't have enough stomach acid to properly digest your food, some of your food sits in your stomach instead of passing through to the small intestine. That partially digested food refluxes back from your stomach up into your esophagus along with some acid, causing a burning sensation, or "heartburn."

Many doctors mistakenly prescribe antacids or proton pump inhibitors to reduce what they believe is excess stomach acid. But frequently the real problem is *not enough* stomach acid. That's why I recommend hydrochloric acid or apple cider vinegar in both phases of the Microbiome Diet so you can be sure to digest your food properly.

ON TO THE SMALL INTESTINE AND THE COLON

From the stomach your food passes to the small intestine. Although the small intestine is coiled neatly within your abdomen, it would be fifteen to twenty feet long if you stretched it out. Within its many folds are billions of microbes, one portion of your microbiome, that help absorb nutrients.

Within your small intestine two remarkable hormones are produced: PYY and GLP-1.

These hormones' names aren't so memorable, but their effects certainly are. GLP-1 increases the amount of time you feel full and satisfied after a meal. So if you wonder why you feel hungry so soon after you eat, insufficient GLP-1 production might well be the answer. If your microbiome isn't balanced, it can't help your small intestine produce this crucial hormone, and you will find, as many of my patients do, that your hunger is raging out of control. GLP-1 also protects the neurons in your brain, helping to prevent dementia and support optimal brain function.

Peptide YY, or PYY for short, is produced in both the small intestine and the colon, and it too responds to the presence of food by making you feel less hungry. It keeps your stomach from emptying too fast so you feel full longer, digest food more efficiently, and absorb more nutrients from what you eat. It might also protect your brain from aluminum, which can cause all sorts of problems.

Another crucial aspect of your small intestine is its epithelial wall, or epithelium. This wall is lined with millions of tiny villi, small projections approximately one millimeter long. The villi wave back and forth, like reeds in a pond, pulling the nutrients from your food in toward your epithelial wall. The cells of that wall pass those nutrients into your bloodstream, which carries them to every part of your body.

Although your epithelial wall has a crucial job to perform, it is only one cell thick. Those cells are constantly dying and being replaced with new cells at a very rapid rate. In fact, the life span of an epithelial cell is only about twenty-four hours. That means you must constantly nourish your body in order to keep your gut wall in good shape.

Stress compromises these cells and makes it difficult for your body to maintain a strong, healthy epithelial wall. That's one way in which stress contributes to leaky gut, which, as we have seen, can lead to weight gain.

The microbiome is also crucial in maintaining the health of those gut walls; in fact, that's one of its main jobs. So when stress compromises your microbiome, your gut walls suffer, and, again, your weight can climb.

After nutrients have been extracted from the food you have eaten, the undigested portion passes into your colon or large intestine. These remains include fiber, the part of fruits, vegetables, and grains that you cannot digest yourself but that provides crucial nourishment for your microbiome. That makes fiber a critical prebiotic.

The microbes in your colon ferment this fiber to produce the short-chain fatty acids, including butyrate and acetate, that are so important for helping you lose weight. The microbes in your colon also produce B vitamins and vitamin K.

We tend to think of ourselves as solid, fixed beings. In fact, however, we are constantly in flux. Red blood cells live for less than four months. Epithelial cells live for less than a day. The bacteria in the microbiome live for only twenty minutes. Our body is in a constant state of flux. It must keep growing and changing or else it will die.

What sustains this extraordinary process of growth and change? Food. We need to constantly take in food so our body has the materials it needs to keep making new cells, repairing bones and muscles and organs, and energizing our brain.

This is why it's so important to eat the food that nourishes all parts of your body, including, of course, the microbiome. It is also why we must protect the process of digestion and not allow it to be compromised by stress, which alters the chemical balance of our bodies and keeps us from getting the nutrients we need. Stress while eating is a big part of the reason so many Americans are both overweight and malnourished.

So save stress for the "fight or flight" reaction, and while you are eating allow yourself to "rest and digest." Your whole body will thank you for it, and you will finally be able to achieve and maintain a healthy weight.

SUPPORT FOR STRESS-FREE EATING

Now I know that many of you are reading this book because you simply want to lose some excess weight. You haven't necessarily signed on for a change in attitude.

Believe me, I get it. But as a scientist and a physician, I have to tell you that changing from stressed eating to stress-free eating will make a major difference in your weight.

So here are a few suggestions that might help you shift from a stressed pattern of eating to a stress-free approach. You don't have to follow them all. Pick one or two you think might work for you, and try to practice at least one each day while you are following the Microbiome Diet. I promise you—it will make a significant difference.

Dos and Don'ts for Stress-Free Eating

- **DON'T eat while working.** Pause and create a space of gratitude, appreciation, and pleasure around your food. (See the meditations below for some suggestions on how to do this.)
- **DON'T skip meals or snacks.** Your body needs to eat every four hours. Skipping meals stresses your system, raises your cortisol levels, and cues your body to store fat.
- **DO chew your food thoroughly.** Try to chew every bite of food at least twenty times before swallowing. This will probably seem like a huge change and, at first, almost impossible to do. But give it a try—you will be amazed at how much more you enjoy your meals *and* how much easier weight loss becomes!
- **DO savor your food.** In a food-abundant culture it is easy to take food for granted. But having food available to satisfy your hunger is actually a great privilege. Enjoying the taste, texture, and aroma of every bite you eat helps you benefit from the "French paradox" and makes losing weight easier.
- 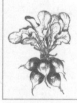**DO focus on your food or else eat food in good company.** Studies show that when people eat while watching TV they tend to eat more, simply because they are not paying attention. Eat in a way in which either food or communing with loved ones becomes the main focus of the meal. Your stress response will subside and your weight will drop.

SAVOR EVERY BITE

Experiment with focused eating by devoting one entire meal to simply savoring your food. Choose a quiet, peaceful atmosphere in which to eat, perhaps with soft background music playing. Light a candle. Set a beautiful place for yourself. Put flowers on the table in a nice vase or choose other ornaments that give you pleasure to look at.

When you eat, take your time. Chew every bite at least twenty times. After you have done this exercise once or twice chew every bite at least thirty times. See how long you can hold each bite of food inside your mouth. See how much flavor, aroma, texture, and warmth or coolness you can get from every molecule of food.

GIVE THANKS

Whatever your cultural background or current beliefs, you can benefit greatly from taking a moment to appreciate the food you are about to eat. If you practice a religious tradition, you can turn to one of the "graces" or "blessings" in that tradition. Otherwise, simply focus on everything needed to bring this food to your plate: the people who planted it, harvested it, shipped it, and sold it to you and the soil and water and nutrients and bacteria that enabled the food to grow. If you are eating meat, acknowledge the creature that gave its life so you can nourish yourself. Take a moment to feel grateful for everything that came together so you can enjoy this meal.

If "gratitude" feels too sentimental, focus instead on awareness and acknowledgment. By eating the food in front of you, you are taking your place in a web of relationships—with other humans, with plants and animals, with this planet's sun, oceans, and soil. Feel your connection to this larger network and then think about the uses to which you will put the food you are about to consume. Pausing to envision these relationships and thinking about your own contribution to others will have a significant effect on your stress response, your digestion, and your weight.

APPRECIATE YOUR MICROBIOME!

As you look at the food you are about to eat think of the microbiome that will soon be helping you digest it. Instead of asking only how good a certain food looks or imagining how delicious it will taste, ask yourself, "Will this food be healthy for me? Is it going to contribute to an improvement in my gut? Will it nourish and balance my microbiome?"

WHEN YOU HAVE TO EAT ON THE RUN

Even if you sometimes have to eat in stressful circumstances—while working, with people you find difficult, or within a very short time—you can take control of your digestive process and destress your eating in less than sixty seconds. Before you take your first bite, pause, take a deep breath, exhale slowly, and do one of the following:

- Picture where the food came from and give a quick thanks to the people, animals, plants, and aspects of nature that created this meal for you.
- Think about what you are going to do with the energy you get from this food. Consecrate the food to a good purpose or to the service of someone you love.
- Inhale on a slow count of four, hold your breath for four counts, and then exhale slowly on eight counts. Exhaling on a count twice as long as your inhale automatically engages your parasympathetic nervous system.
- Envision your sympathetic nervous system—your "fight or flight" response—that currently has you in its grip. Thank your body for giving you such a great way to respond to stress, but instruct it to switch momentarily to the parasympathetic nervous system, which governs the "rest or digest" response. Tell your body, "You can return to the sympathetic nervous system when I am done eating, but for optimal digestion I want the parasympathetic nervous system to remain in control while I am eating."

Although you might not be used to looking at food in this way, remember all those animal studies from Chapter 7. Eating when you feel stressed cues your body to hold onto fat, and eating when you feel relaxed cues your body to burn fat. Put your body into a fat-burning mood by finding ways to shift quickly and efficiently from "fight or flight" to "rest and digest." It will make a significant difference to your gut, your health, and your weight.

FINDING MEANING AT THE TABLE

For good or ill, we humans have a complicated relationship to food. Unlike animals—even stressed ones!—we eat when we are not hungry, we create foods that are not healthy for us, and we gobble our food while we drive, while we watch TV, and while we work.

Rituals and customs around food have many sources and serve many purposes, but as a physician, I am struck that one of their great benefits is to help us switch from the sympathetic to the parasympathetic nervous system, from "fight or flight" to "rest and digest." I am also struck by the way they help us find meaning in the act of eating. I am convinced that the need for meaning is one of the most profound of all human needs.

I've seen it with thousands of patients over the years: when food and meaning come together people often lose weight. When my patients take time to enjoy each bite, they eat less because they are giving their leptin-based "fullness reaction" time to kick in. When my patients eat in an atmosphere of connectedness and love, they digest better and burn more fat because they are giving their digestive systems optimal support and avoiding the cortisol-based stress response that cues their bodies for fat storage.

If we create meaning in every moment we eat, we will go a long way toward freeing ourselves from our cravings. Slowly but surely we will find ourselves desiring only the food that truly satisfies our bodies and helps us on our journey toward overall health and wellness.

nine

CREATING THE METABOLISM OF A THIN PERSON

W HEN MY PATIENT SUSANNAH WALKED INTO MY OFFICE HER FIRST words were to tell me how hopeless she felt.

"I've come here because I know you helped my friend Nikki lose weight," she said. "And she said your diet worked after she'd spent years trying all the others. She made me promise to at least give you a try. But I have to be honest—I don't think it will help."

I asked Susannah why she was so pessimistic. Her answer didn't surprise me because it was something I had heard from many other patients over the years.

"Look," she said, "everybody in my family is fat. My parents are both very overweight. My sister weighs even more than I do, and even though my brother works out all the time, he's built like a linebacker—he's just huge. My grandparents are heavy, and so is everybody on both sides of my family. It's just how we're built. I think we've all got fat genes, and there's just nothing we can do about it."

Many of my patients are convinced there is a genetic component to their difficulties with weight, and I'm not necessarily inclined to doubt them. We know our genes have a lot to say about our body size and shape, and this can certainly have a big effect on our metabolism.

But, as I told Susannah, genes are only a part of the story—and not even the most important part.

First, as we have seen in previous chapters, the budding science of epigenetics shows us we can have an enormous impact on the way our genes express themselves. If you have a genetic predisposition toward diabetes, for example, you can "turn down the volume" on those genes by avoiding sweet or starchy foods, getting sufficient exercise, and, of course, supporting your microbiome.

Likewise, if you have a genetic predisposition toward weight gain, you can "turn down the volume" on those genes by boosting your metabolism. Once you support your microbiome, your metabolism will automatically rev up.

But even more excitingly, I explained to Susannah, we don't have to rely only on *our* genes alone; the genes of our microbiome can also help us reshape our genetic destiny.

After all, only a tiny portion of the genetic material within our bodies belongs to us. The genes of our microbiome outnumber ours by 150 to 1. When we reshape *their* genetic composition, we reshape our own ability to lose weight. Do you want to have a metabolism like that thin friend of yours who eats a few desserts each month and still maintains her healthy weight? Supporting your microbiome is the key. Its genes can help you transform your own.

HOW THE MICROBIOME DIET RESHAPES YOUR GENES

One way to affect the genetic composition of our microbiome, I told Susannah, is by eating the foods that support friendly bacteria and avoiding foods that support unfriendly bacteria. The wrong foods can inflame your system within about five hours, whereas the right foods can create an equally rapid healthy response.

Why does diet work so quickly to reshape your microbiome? Because the life span of a bacterial microbe is only about twenty minutes. Five hours are the equivalent of fifteen microbial lifetimes, or, in human terms, more than a thousand years. In that time the microbial population can shift from unfriendly to friendly, or vice versa.

To make matters even better, the organisms in your microbiome can actually exchange genes with one another. This gives them an extraordinary flexibility—for their genome and also for yours.

And so, I told Susannah, the Microbiome Diet would not only help her lose weight; it would also allow her to re-create her genetic destiny. She could transform her entire metabolism, leaving behind the family metabolism and becoming someone whose body worked quite differently. Instead of being someone who seemingly only had to look at food to gain weight, Susannah could have the metabolism of her much-envied friends, someone who could maintain only 70 percent compliance without ever gaining weight.

Susannah was understandably skeptical. But she agreed to give the Microbiome Diet a try. She followed Phase 1 to the letter, avoiding the sugar, reactive foods, grains, and legumes that might feed unhealthy bacteria while she also loaded up on the healing foods that support healthy bacteria.

To Susannah's astonishment, she lost seven pounds in three weeks—more than she had ever been able to lose on previous diets. Then, when she began Phase 2, she was torn. She looked forward to the greater variety of foods that I prescribe for Phase 2, but she was somewhat nervous about the idea of adhering to the plan only 90 percent of the time.

"Are you *sure* I can eat whatever I want 10 percent of the time?" she asked. "I can't believe I won't just gain everything back right away."

"Well, I don't exactly want you eating *whatever* you want," I said. "I would prefer you permanently avoid trans fats and hydrogenated fats because they are so unhealthy. Although it's not the end of the world if you have them once every few months, ideally you would choose other foods for your 10 percent. But, yes, you're safe to indulge 10 percent of the time. Your metabolism is different now—you have really altered your genetic destiny! Why don't you experiment and see how it goes. If you find you're gaining weight or failing to lose it, you can always go back to a stricter regime."

The next time I saw Susannah she had completed the four weeks of Phase 2 and was ready to move on to Phase 3. She had continued to lose weight, slowly and steadily, and was excited about this new way of eating, which left her feeling full, satisfied, and energized. Her skin was glowing, her hair was thicker than before, and, she told me, "I haven't gotten a cold all winter, which is not at all like me!"

All of these side effects, I told her, were testimony to how profoundly an altered microbiome can transform your body, your metabolism, and your weight.

RESETTING YOUR METABOLISM BY SUPPORTING YOUR THYROID

One of the reasons people often gain weight or have a hard time losing it is because of insufficient thyroid hormone. Your body needs thyroid hormone to help regulate your metabolism, promote regular elimination, and support your hair, nails, and skin.

Your thyroid gland makes two types of hormone, known as T3 and T4. Only about 10 or 20 percent of what your gland produces is T3, the active form of thyroid hormone. The rest is T4, an inactive hormone that must be converted to T3 before it can have any effect on your body.

About 20 percent of your T4 is converted into T3 within your intestinal tract, but only when you have a healthy microbiome. So when the Microbiome Diet rebalances your microbiome it also reboots your thyroid production.

Another portion of T4 is converted in your liver. So if your liver isn't functioning properly, you also end up low in the active T3 form of thyroid hormone. And why might your liver fail to function at optimal levels? The culprit is, once again, inflammation.

So once again an imbalanced microbiome creates a vicious circle:

imbalanced microbiome	→	unhealthy gut	→	insufficient thyroid conversion	→	sluggish metabolism and weight gain
imbalanced microbiome	→	stressed liver	→	insufficient thyroid conversion	→	sluggish metabolism and weight gain

Conversely, a balanced microbiome creates a virtuous circle:

balanced microbiome	→	healthy gut	→	sufficient thyroid conversion	→	balanced metabolism and healthy weight
balanced microbiome	→	healthy liver	→	sufficient thyroid conversion	→	balanced metabolism and healthy weight

THE MICROBIOME AND AUTOIMMUNE CONDITIONS

Nishi was one of the many patients who come to me when other physicians were not able to determine a diagnosis. She was about forty pounds overweight—weight that she had been gaining steadily over the past five or six years—but to her, the weight was secondary. She was far more concerned about joint pain, fatigue, and disturbingly high readings for CRP and Interleukin-6, two classic markers of inflammation.

High CRP readings put Nishi at risk for heart disease, and the joint pain and fatigue suggested she had some kind of autoimmune condition, perhaps rheumatoid arthritis. But Nishi did not fit the classic profile of rheumatoid arthritis.

Nishi had read that many people with autoimmune condition are gluten-sensitive, so she had cut gluten completely out of her diet. However, she told me, that dietary change had basically made no difference in her condition. In fact, when I ran a complete gluten panel on Nishi, no sensitivities showed up. So what was causing her symptoms?

I have seen many people with situations like Nishi's—apparently unrelated symptoms that don't quite fit the profile of recognized diseases along with mysterious and frustrating weight gain. I began giving Nishi the supplements I usually prescribe to support the microbiome: probiotics, prebiotics, and short-chain fatty acids, including butyrate. I had her follow the Microbiome Diet, loading up on healing foods. I explained the way stress impairs the microbiome and the digestive process, and I gave her my suggestions for stress-free eating.

As I said, Nishi was not even concerned with weight loss. Yet when she returned to me three weeks after our initial visit not only had her symptoms abated, but she had also lost eight pounds. In Phase 2 of the Microbiome Diet she went on to lose another twenty pounds, even as her energy returned, her inflammatory markers went down, and her joint pain disappeared.

A great deal of evidence suggests that healing the digestive system can help people with autoimmune conditions, including rheumatoid arthritis, lupus, multiple sclerosis, fibromyalgia, and Hashimoto's thyroiditis. No research has specifically linked the microbiome with these conditions, but recall that 70 percent of the immune system lies just below the epithelial wall and that the microbiome helps to rebuild that wall. Because the microbiome also helps to support digestive health, I believe there is a connection. I have also seen in many patients how healing the microbiome eases the symptoms of autoimmune disorders. If effortless weight loss is another side effect, so much the better!

THE METABOLISM OF A THIN PERSON

How many times have you looked at a friend or coworker who seemed able to eat whatever they wanted and still remain at a healthy weight? I'm not talking about people who exercise maniacally or who binge and starve. I'm talking about people who seem to eat in a healthy, relaxed way and then, every so often, indulge.

What enables these seemingly blessed people to maintain their healthy weights while periodically—even frequently—indulging? Yes, to some extent, genes are involved, but, as we saw with Susannah, our genetic destiny can be extraordinarily malleable.

My belief is that the blessed people with the robust metabolisms have well-balanced microbiomes that they support by eating the healing foods featured on the Microbiome Diet while avoiding, by and large, starchy foods, too much sugar, and unhealthy fats. Yes, every so often they might indulge. But their healthy microbiomes give them that leeway. You can have that leeway too.

The true goal of the Microbiome Diet is a body so restored to health that you can follow its lead, letting your body tell you when it's hungry, what kind of food its needs, and what circumstances allow you to make the most of every meal. As you enter Phase 2 of this healing diet I invite you to enjoy every bite you eat, secure in the knowledge that you can trust your microbiome to keep your weight on track.

PART IV

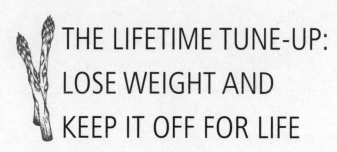

THE LIFETIME TUNE-UP:
LOSE WEIGHT AND
KEEP IT OFF FOR LIFE

ten

TOWARD A HEALTHY FUTURE

Once you have finished with Phases 1 and 2 of the Microbiome Diet your microbiome should be in a healthy, balanced state. I hope you have also been able to develop a new relationship to food, in which you feel free of cravings yet able to enjoy your meals to the utmost!

As a result Phase 3 of the Microbiome Diet has no meal plans. By the time you reach Phase 3 you know how to support your microbiome. You have given your body a chance to free itself of cravings and hormonal imbalances. Now you know what your body really needs, and you probably have begun to crave those foods while losing interest in the others.

I have given you the figure 70 percent compliance as a general guideline, which means that of the thirty-five meals and snacks you eat during the week, about ten of them can include foods I have been asking you to avoid. I would counsel you to continue to avoid hydrogenated and trans fats because they are so bad for you as well as to avoid GMOs (for more on GMOs, see pages 154–155). I also strongly encourage you to keep loading up on fermented foods and healing foods as well as to keep taking your supplements and probiotics. When you turn to Phase 3 in the following section you will find a few more guidelines as well.

Finally, I want you to continue in your commitment to stress-free eating, whether you are indulging in a scoop of ice cream or eating a microbiome-friendly portion of kimchee! Stress-free eating is both more pleasurable and more healthy than eating on the run, so ideally you will eat that way 100 percent of the time. Stress-free eating manifests your pleasure and appreciation in the food you eat, allowing your body to "rest and digest" rather than "fight or flee." It is crucial for maintaining both a healthy microbiome and a healthy weight.

Other than that, you now have more leeway in your food choices, because now your body is your own best guide. You know which foods give you pleasure, you know how much you need to eat before you have had enough, and you know how your body feels after a healthy meal. Now you are able to listen to your body and to your microbiome.

What does this mean for day-to-day food choices? It means when you get the signals telling you that you'd like some sautéed onions in your omelet or that you'd really love some fresh blueberries or that you can't wait to sip some warm, comforting chicken-bone soup, you can trust those signals and respond. And when you get the signal telling you that "It's probably fine to have a few French fries" or "Today it's okay to indulge in a dessert," you can listen to those signals also.

If you continue to listen to your body, you will also hear signals steering you away from unhealthy choices. Your body or your microbiome might lead you to say to yourself, "I don't really want a starchy snack—I'd rather have something fresh, instead!" or "Sugar really doesn't appeal to me today—I've had two desserts already this week, and I'm kind of sugared out."

Remember, if you have to take antibiotics, make sure you are also taking probiotics. And if you end up bingeing or going off the diet significantly, go back to Phase 1 and remain on it until you feel healthy and clear again.

Now that you have this new relationship to food, I'd like to share with you some of the bigger issues behind the Microbiome Diet, some of the deeper ideas that have driven my approach to diet, food, and health.

THE BIG PICTURE: WHAT'S BEHIND
THE OBESITY EPIDEMIC?

I'll be honest: even though I have had lots of success in helping my patients lose weight, I always resisted writing a book about weight loss. For many years it seemed that most of the diets out there had little to do with the real core issues of health, and I couldn't see where my own ideas would fit in. To me, weight loss and health are not two separate issues—they are one and the same. But for a long time diet books seemed to focus only on weight loss, ignoring the deeper concerns.

Over the past few years, however, many diet book authors have taken a more integrated approach, addressing not only weight loss but also the larger issues of what the body needs. Step by step, the best diet books began to approach the core issues for weight loss and health.

Some books, for example, focused on inflammation. Others focused on food sensitivities, leaky gut, and intestinal health. Still, none of these approaches offered us sufficient power to counteract the obesity epidemic, which continued to skyrocket even while diet books crowded the shelves. The obesity epidemic was still too powerful for us because we didn't really understand why it was happening. Why was there such a dramatic increase in insulin resistance? Why was there such an explosion in food sensitivities? Why were so many people claiming that even when they ate carefully and exercised regularly they still saw their weight creeping up and up and up?

I simply did not believe that willpower was at the root of this epidemic. It made no sense to me that for thousands of years people maintained relatively healthy weights without benefit of diet books or diet plans, and then suddenly they began caving in to a mindless desire to overeat. For thousands of years on this planet we humans have had the biological capacity for leaky gut, intestinal distress, insulin resistance, and inflammation. Yet these conditions had never before skyrocketed out of control—and now, suddenly, they were. What had changed?

I believe attacks on the microbiome—from toxins, antibiotics, unhealthy foods, and stress—are the cause of the current obesity epidemic. The microbiome is the ultimate cause behind all the other causes spoken about in previous diet books. Yes, insulin resistance causes weight gain, but an imbalanced microbiome is the real culprit behind insulin resistance. Yes, inflammation and leptin resistance create weight gain, but an imbalanced microbiome is driving that inflammation. Yes, leaky gut and food sensitivities create weight gain, but an imbalanced microbiome is largely responsible for that leaky gut. Yes, gluten in its new, hybridized, de-aminized, and omnipresent forms helps to create leaky gut, weight gain, and a host of other symptoms, but an imbalanced microbiome is responsible for the weakened gut walls that enable gluten to have such a potent effect.

With such pioneering researchers as Martin J. Blaser, I believe attacks on the microbiome are behind the obesity epidemic. Luckily, now that we understand the problem, we can solve it. Supporting the microbiome, through individual diet as well as social changes in our ecology, will enable us to resolve the crisis.

THE MICROBIOME AND OUR CURRENT HEALTH CRISIS

Physicians today are faced with a tremendous paradox. On the one hand, we have achieved vastly increased life expectancy and have significantly extended the quality of life for people as they age. When I was a child, sixty was considered old. Now we have sixty-year-olds who jog three miles a day, found brand-new businesses or embark on new careers, and begin new romances or rekindle longstanding marriages. These are the victories of modern medicine and modern nutrition, the fruits of our protein-rich diet, our access to antibiotics, and other medical miracles.

On the other hand, we have an increase in allergies, autoimmune conditions, cancers, and diabetes. Metabolic syndrome—obesity, high blood pressure, and insulin resistance—is on the rise.

In my opinion the loss of microbial diversity is behind not only the obesity epidemic but also the allergic epidemic, the explosion in autoimmune conditions, the rise in cancer, and pretty much every other first-world medical crisis. Just as the destruction of the rain forests, climate change, oil spills, and the proliferation of industrial chemicals threaten the outer ecology of our planet, so does the loss of diversity in the microbiome threaten our inner ecology.

Just as the microbiome is behind our obesity epidemic, I believe it is at the root of skyrocketing rates of depression, anxiety, and other emotional and cognitive disorders. These are complex problems with many causes, but an imbalanced microbiome and an unhealthy digestive system make it nearly impossible for the brain to function properly. Heal the gut, balance the microbiome, and you have a much greater chance of thinking clearly, feeling optimistic, and enjoying the energy and vitality that is your birthright.

Throughout this book we have seen how the microbiome affects many of the body's systems. Here is a summary that makes it dramatically clear just how deeply the microbiome is involved with our overall health:

OUR INNER AND OUTER ECOLOGIES

Why, then, are we all experiencing such microbial distress? What has so disrupted our inner ecology?

For the answer, I believe we must look toward the outer ecology. Our food, water, and air are full of toxins and pollutants that disrupt our microbiome, stress our immune system, and burden our gastrointestinal tract.

One category of toxins is known as *endocrine disrupters*, or *xenoestrogens*. This is a class of chemicals that mimic the effects of estrogen, creating a hormonal imbalance that, among other things, disrupts our microbiome as well.

RESULTS OF AN UNBALANCED MICROBIOME

Cognitive and Emotional Issues
aggressive behavior
anxiety
autism
brain fog
confusion
dementia
depression
fuzzy thinking
inability to regulate emotions
mood swings
neurodevelopmental disorders
poor memory
sensory disorders

Digestive Issues
bloating
constipation
Crohn's disease
diarrhea
gas
intestinal pain
irritable bowel syndrome
ulcerative colitis

Immune Issues
autoimmune disorders, including Hashimoto's thyroiditis,
    multiple sclerosis, rheutamoid arthritis, lupus,
    fibromyalgia, and Sjogren's syndrome
decreased immune function

Endocrine Disorders
estrogen-progesterone disorders
hypothyroidism
polycystic ovarian syndrome

Metabolic Disorders
diabetes
insulin resistance
metabolic syndrome

Dermatological Disorders

acne

eczema

other skin rashes

psoriasis

Other Symptoms and Disorders

bedwetting

cancer

cardiovascular disorders

hair loss

joint pain

loss of bone density

muscle pain

osteoporosis

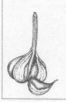

It's not only the antibiotics we take ourselves that can wreak havoc on our gut health; as we have seen, most of the beef, milk, cheese, yogurt, chicken, eggs, turkey, lamb, and pork we consume is also loaded with antibiotics. These powerful medications are given either to protect the animals from the diseases that arise when they are raised in close, unsanitary quarters or administered specifically with the intent of fattening them up.

In addition, industrial chemicals used in manufacturing make their way into our groundwater, our soil, and our air, and these toxins further challenge our intestinal health. As we have seen, what disrupts the gut disrupts the immune system as well. First, our immune system is overwhelmed by having to protect us against this onslaught of toxic attackers. Then it is baffled by the presence of toxins that it's never seen before.

So we in effect train our immune system to "go crazy" and then we hand it a gun. It's powerful, it's out of control, and it's overwhelmed with potential targets. No wonder our immune systems begin attacking our own cells, healthy foods, or harmless specks of dust, as happens to people with asthma and related allergies. No wonder food sensitivities and allergies are on the rise while our bodies cope with system-wide inflammation. And no wonder this extraordinary amount of physical stress, not to mention the psychological stressors of modern life, make the inflammation worse and cue our bodies to store fat.

To make matters worse, we are also being exposed to genetically modified organisms, or GMOs. Most of the corn, soy, canola, potatoes, and cotton in the United States have been genetically modified and so have many vegetables and fruits. If we eat processed foods, we are likely getting small doses of genetically modified corn and soy in just about every bite we take.

Simply scrambling the genes is bad enough, but sometimes the genetic modification includes sequencing toxins right into the food. Corn, for example, is modified with a toxin that is supposed to keep the insects away. But traces of those toxins have turned up in mothers' breast milk. Because most corn is used to feed cattle, it's possible that even if the careful mother made every effort to avoid GMOs, she absorbed the GMO-related toxins through seemingly innocent meat or milk.

Another goal of genetically engineering crops is to make them tolerant to glyphosate, a chemical used in herbicides. That way farmers can spray their crops with glyphosate, kill the weeds, and leave the crops standing. Corn, soybeans, canola, cotton, sugar beets, and alfalfa have all been modified in this way.

But glyphosate wreaks havoc on the microbiome. What effect must it have on our inner ecology to consume food that has been treated, repeatedly, with this chemical or to eat the products of animals who have been fed with glyphosate-coated corn or soy?

Most chilling of all is the prospect of the genetic alterations in the crops somehow affecting the genetic composition of the microbiome and, through our microbiome, our own genes. Industry spokespeople insist this isn't possible, but we do have some chilling evidence at hand. A 2004 study reported by the US National Academy of Sciences found that parts of the altered gene in genetically modified soy could be transferred into the DNA of microbial bacteria.

So what happens if these altered genes are not eliminated with our waste products as genetic engineers assure us they will be? What happens if instead these altered genes remain in our intestinal tract and become part of our microbiome? What might be the effect on our digestive or our immune systems?

According to Dr. Jack Heinemann, professor of genetics and molecular biology at the University of Canterbury in New Zealand, we can believe "in no reasonable uncertainty that genetically modified plant material can transfer to animals exposed to genetically modified feed in their diets or environment, and that there can be a residual difference in animals or animal product as a result of exposure to genetically modified food."

In other words, altered genes can be transferred into our microbiome, and they can alter *us* as a result.

So in the face of all these assaults—the endocrine disrupters, toxins, and altered genes—along with the profusion of antibiotics, our microbiome is losing its diversity at an alarming rate. What was once a beautiful lush forest has now become a few skeletal remains. If you picture the smoking ruins that hang on after a forest fire, that should give you some idea of how devastated our microbiome has become.

Luckily, there is a solution. If we repair the ecological devastation in our outer world and support the microbiome within us, we can bring that lush forest back to life. Every step we take to nourish our microbiome adds to the energy, optimism, and vitality we bring to this crucial ecological renewal.

RE-EMPOWERMENT

It can feel terribly disempowering to envision the extent to which our global ecology is in distress. But I don't want to leave you feeling defeated, particularly because, as we saw in Chapter 7, the defeat reaction is characterized by insulin resistance, abnormal cholesterol metabolism, retention of abdominal fat, and other factors that slow your metabolism and increase your weight.

Instead, I want to do two things. I want you to feel validated in your sense that you are indeed up against powerful forces that are out of your control—the food industry, which floods the market with unhealthy choices; industrial polluters, who overwhelm your world with toxins and endocrine disrupters; the corporations that develop, grow, and sell genetically modified products; and the government that permits and sometimes even encourages these practices. You aren't making it up: there really are powerful forces arrayed against you, making it more difficult for you to regain control of your health and lose your unwanted weight.

And I want you to remember that you *are* a powerful being, capable of cleaning up your inner ecology and joining with others to clean up our outer ecology. Reconnecting with your body and your microbiome—that extraordinary intelligence within you—can restore your health, rebalance your immune system, and rejuvenate your gastrointestinal tract. It can also return you to a healthy weight. Although you are up against powerful forces, you can succeed, especially now that you are armed with the power and knowledge of the Microbiome Diet. When you reconnect to the collective intelligence of your microbiome, when you support your inner ecology, and when you learn how to listen to your body and hear what it needs, you will be empowered to make the choices that boost your metabolism and bring you to a healthy weight. Trillions of microorganisms within your brain, gut, and cells are ready to help you succeed—if you only give them the nourishment they need.

THE MICROBIOME BANQUET

As I was writing this book I chanced across a fascinating article with a very powerful title: "Meaning Is Healthier Than Happiness." Published by Emily Esfahani Smith in the online edition of the *Atlantic*, the article shared the results of a new study from the *Proceedings of the National Academy of Sciences*. Using the imaging from a functional MRI, the researchers explored what happens on a genetic level in various conditions: happy, but with little sense of meaning, and having a deep sense of meaning. Meaning, in this study, was defined as "an orientation to something bigger than the self."

What the researchers found was that genetic expression was healthier in the group of people who lived with a deep sense of meaning. Both people who faced chronic adversity and those who felt happy without much meaning seemed to have immune systems keyed toward producing more inflammation. And, as we have seen, inflammation is a risk factor for a wide variety of diseases and, most significantly, for weight gain.

So as you begin the Microbiome Diet I would like to invite you to recommit to your own search for meaning. In my experience we can find profound meaning in our food, which connects us to the plants and animals of this planet; the soil, air, and water needed to nourish that food; and the human community whose labor was needed to grow our food and transport it to us.

We can also find meaning within our own bodies. I am struck, for example, that our intestinal tract needs glutamine to function, but its first action, always, is to metabolize the glucose the rest of the body needs. In that sense, our own digestive system is selfless, finding its own meaning by operating for the good of the whole. When we connect to our bodies we connect to that principle as well, learning to find meaning in what we give to others as well as in what we receive from them.

And, of course, we can find profound meaning in our microbiome. The collective intelligence of the microbiome always places the whole above the individual. Fascinating research has shown how microscopic organisms—with life spans of less than twenty minutes—collectively decide which bacteria shall be sacrificed for the good of the whole, exchange genetic material, and mediate between their own needs and those of their human host.

Furthermore I believe that collective spirit extends from the microbiome to us. Although they feed on the food we give them, they spend the vast majority of their energy not on their own survival but on ours. They are a model of how true giving and putting the welfare of the whole above our own individual needs is actually the path to fulfillment.

How can we carry forth that meaning in our daily act of eating? We can make every meal a banquet, for ourselves and those whom we invite—our human guests and our microbial guests as well. We can become selfless givers who understand that love and generosity are healing emotions, supporting the immune system, reducing inflammation, and counteracting the stress that causes us to gain unhealthy weight. We can feel the love inherent in the food we eat, appreciating its sensual pleasures and promising to put the energy it gives us to good use.

We can also remember that food is not a commodity and our bodies are not machines. That approach to food has produced an outer ecology that is full of GMOs and high-fructose corn syrup, industrial farms and antibiotic-laden animals that make us fat by the same means that their owners made them fat. Treating food in that way does not help us create true health, and it does not make us feel like the powerful, loving, interconnected beings we truly are.

Rather, we can view food as a vital relationship that literally brings us into the flow of life, involving us with other living creatures, with nature itself, and with our planet. Feeling ourselves in the flow of life, knowing we are a vital part of the whole, and cherishing both the inner and the outer ecologies—that is the road to health, empowerment, and self-love, wherever we are on our weight loss journey.

So here's to you as you host your own microbiome banquet! The ultimate goal of the Microbiome Diet is to help you enter the true flow of life.

PART V

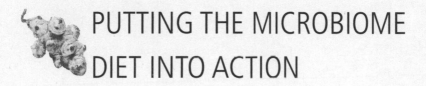PUTTING THE MICROBIOME
DIET INTO ACTION

eleven

YOUR MICROBIOME SUPERFOODS

The principles of the Microbiome Diet are simple:

- Load up on the foods that heal your gut and support your microbiome.
- Avoid the foods that challenge your gut and imbalance your microbiome.

As we have seen, healing your gut and supporting your microbiome will automatically lead to healthy weight loss. When your gut is in optimal condition and your microbiome is balanced, your body will naturally find and remain at its healthy weight.

Of course, you will also enjoy a wide variety of fresh fruits and vegetables, healthy fats, and lean proteins. But our focus will be on the Microbiome Superfoods, Superspices, and Supersupplements—foods, spices, and supplements that have an extraordinary ability to support your microbiome, heal your gut, and enable weight loss. Let me introduce you to these Superfoods so you can feel as enthusiastic about them as I do.

YOUR MICROBIOME SUPERFOODS

Natural probiotics, which replenish your microbiome with additional healthy bacteria

- Fermented vegetables, such as sauerkraut and kimchee
- Fermented dairy products, such as kefir and yogurt made from sheep's or goat's milk

Natural prebiotics, which nourish the healthy bacteria already in your microbiome

- Asparagus
- Carrots
- Garlic
- Jerusalem artichoke
- Jicama
- Leeks
- Onions
- Radishes
- Tomatoes

YOUR MICROBIOME SUPERSPICES

- Cinnamon, which balances blood sugar and, therefore, insulin, helping to prevent insulin resistance and thereby cuing your body to burn fat rather than store it
- Turmeric, a natural anti-inflammatory that helps heal the gut, support the microbiome, and promote good brain function

YOUR MICROBIOME SUPERSUPPLEMENTS

NOTE: If you are taking medication of any kind, please check with your health care provider before taking supplements so as to ensure there are no contraindications or adverse side effects.

To REMOVE unhealthy bacteria from your intestines

- Berberine
- Caprylic acid
- Garlic
- Grapefruit seed extract
- Oregano Oil
- Wormwood

To REPLACE stomach acid and digestive enzymes

- Hydrochloric Acid
- Amylase, which digests starches
- Apple cider vinegar
- DPP 41V, which helps digest gluten and casein (milk protein)
- Lipase, which digests fat
- Protease, which digests protein

To REINOCULATE with probiotics and prebiotics

- A good probiotic:
  - Contains many diverse species
  - Contains at least these three types of *Lactobacillus*: *acidophilus*, *rameneses*, *planataris*
  - Contains different types of *Bifidobacter*
  - A bonus is if it contains *Acidophilus reuterii*
  - Should contain between 50 billion and 200 billion bacteria—the more, the better.
- Most probiotics do not contain *Acidophilus gasseri*, but it has shown to be extremely effective in promoting weight loss. You can buy it separately (see Resources) or buy a probiotic that contains it (see Resources).
- Prebiotics
  - Arabinogalactans
  - Cal-mag butyrate
  - Inulin powder

To REPAIR the gut wall

- Carnosine
- DGL (diglycerinated licorice)
- Glutamine
- Marshmallow
- N-acetyl glucosamine
- Quercitin
- Slippery Elm
- Zinc

For weight loss

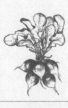

- Garcinia mangostana
- Green Coffee Bean extract
- Irvingia (African mango)
- Meratrim
- Sphaeranthus indicus

THE NEXT GENERATION OF SUPERFOODS

The term "superfood" first became popular several years ago. It was never a scientific designation but more of a quick and easy way for journalists writing about nutrition to indicate some foods that seemed unusually good for our health.

Specifically, superfoods were supposed to have large quantities of antioxidants, chemicals that reduced oxidative stress. Even though oxygen is vital to the body's functioning, it also ages our cells. Antioxidants help our cells fight back, renewing and revitalizing our bodies in the face of the aging process. So the foods that seemed high in antioxidants were dubbed "superfoods."

Unfortunately, it's not that simple. What matters more than the nutrients themselves is whether our bodies can absorb and make use of them. If our microbiome is unbalanced and our gut is in distress, we can consume huge quantities of vitamins, minerals, and antioxidants without ever making a real difference to our health. We need a healthy gut to actually absorb the antioxidants we consume so these chemicals actually work to support our cells. We need a balanced microbiome to keep our gut healthy as well as to make use of the antioxidants, vitamins, and minerals we consume.

So on the Microbiome Diet I have created what I believe is the next generation of superfoods—the Microbiome Superfoods, Superspices, and Supersupplements. These are the foods, spices, and supplements that help heal our gut and balance our microbiome. These Microbiome Superfoods are crucial for absorbing the vitamins, minerals, and antioxidants we consume. They are also a critical aspect of achieving and maintaining a healthy weight.

You can't mimic the benefits of these Microbiome Superfoods by taking supplements. In each Microbiome Superfood nature has created a unique blend of nutrients, antioxidants, anti-inflammatories, and prebiotics—a special combination that works in fellowship to heal our gut, nourish our microbiome, and boost our general health. No nutritionist, scientist, or physician can do as good a job as nature itself has done. And no weight loss specialist could duplicate this job either.

Because of their effects on our microbiome and intestinal tract, these Microbiome Superfoods are crucial elements in weight loss.

The first two phases of the Microbiome Diet are full of these Microbiome Superfoods. By the time you reach Phase 3 I hope you will be used to loading up your diet with these extraordinary foods. To me, they embody the teachings of Hippocrates, the ancient founder of Western medicine, who said many centuries ago, "Let food be your medicine and medicine be your food."

FERMENTED FOODS: NATURAL PROBIOTICS

Fermented foods contain live bacteria that function as natural probiotics—a food-based way to replenish the healthy bacteria in your microbiome. Significantly, every culture in the world seems to have its own fermented foods, suggesting how crucial they are to our health.

I want you to appreciate how traditional cultures have long understood our need to consume fermented foods, so here's a chart that offers a brief sampling of fermented foods around the world. Fermented foods take many forms: pastes, seasonings, condiments, curries, stews, pickles, and even candy. They can be fried or boiled or sometimes candied, and they can be eaten in main dishes, side dishes, salads, or desserts. Fermented drinks can be alcoholic, such as beer and wine, or nonalcoholic, such as certain teas, vinegar-based drinks, or buttermilk. Most of these foods won't appear on the Microbiome Diet, but the universal consumption of fermented foods makes it crystal clear how important this type of food is in any human diet.

Sadly, Western fast foods and packaged foods are wiping out traditional food cultures, and the skills of fermenting food—once known to every household—are being lost. I think this is one of the causes of the worldwide obesity epidemic, which appears in any country where the modern Western diet takes hold. As we have seen, a depleted microbiome leads to weight gain, whereas fermented foods help keep our microbiome balanced and healthy. When we stop eating them our microbiome takes a hit—and weight gain is the result.

Country	Foods
Caucasus	koumiss, a fermented milk drink
China	douchi, a fermented black bean sauce
China, Middle East	kombucha, a fizzy, fermented tea
Russia	kvass, a fizzy beer-like drink made from black or rye bread
Ethiopia/Eritrea	injera, a spongy bread made from fermented teff flour
Ghana	fufu, a fermented product made from cassava, yams, or plantains
Himalayas	bhatti jaanr, fermented rice food-beverage
	gundruk, a fermented leafy vegetable
	kodo ko-jaanr, a fermented millet product
	sinki, a fermented radish
India	dhokla, a steamed food made from fermented rice and chickpeas
	dhosa, a dish of fermented rice and lentils
Japan	miso, fermented soybean paste, used in soups and sauces
	natto, fermented soybean cake
	tempeh, steamed and mashed fermented soybeans
Mexico	pulque, fermented alcoholic beverage made from cactus juice
Nigeria	garri, a fermented product made from cassava
Russia	kvass, a fizzy fermented beer made from black bread or rye bread
South Pacific	poi, fermented taro paste
Thailand	pla ra, fermented fish sauce

Accordingly I have you load up with fermented foods throughout Phases 1 and 2 of the Microbiome Diet, and I hope you will continue this habit when you move into your own Phase 3. The foods I have chosen are the ones most easily available to those of us living in the United States:

- Sauerkraut—a version of fermented cabbage eaten throughout Eastern Europe, Russia, Austria, and Germany
- Kimchee—a Korean version of fermented cabbage, carrots, onions, and garlic
- Fermented vegetables—available ready-made in most stores and online (see Resources), or, if you want to make your own, check out the book *Wild Fermentation: The Flavor, Nutrition, and Craft of Live-Culture Foods* by Sandor Ellix Katz
- Kefir—a fermented milk drink from the north Caucasus (I recommend drinking only sheep's or goat's milk kefir, as that is easier to digest than cow's milk products)
- Yogurt—another type of fermented milk product eaten throughout central and west Asia, India, central Europe, and the Balkans (Again, I recommend focusing on sheep's or goat's milk yogurt. I advise you to avoid the commercial products that are heavily sweetened and have added sugars and fruits.)

What I like about fermented foods is that they turn the whole concept of dieting upside down. Instead of focusing on what you must restrict and remove from your diet, we focus on how you can enrich your diet and improve your health.

Certainly fermented foods have numerous health benefits. Kefir, for example, offers incredible support for your immune system and has traditionally been used to treat tuberculosis and cancer. Kimchee helps lower cholesterol, prevent constipation, and fight colon cancer as well as reduce stress, ease depression, combat osteoarthritis, reduce atherosclerosis, and fight liver disease.

I also love the way fermented foods connect us to the rich history of human food culture over the centuries. Here is where I depart from the Paleo Diet. The Paleo approach seeks to return our food habits to a time before agriculture and the cultivation of domestic animals so we eliminate permanently all grains, legumes, and dairy products. The diet has many good features and may have helped some people improve their weight and health, but I cannot go along with a philosophy that seeks to erase the millennia of human development that has taken place since the Paleolithic Era.

We humans live not just in the world of our bodies but also in the worlds of culture and emotion. The food traditions we have developed speak deeply to us on many levels, and our challenge now is to find a healthy way to incorporate those traditions, not simply to bypass them. Our food choices should spring from a blend of intuition, culture, art, and science. Yes, we need to listen to the latest scientific findings, but we also need to appreciate the centuries that it took for our ancestors to perfect the cultivation of yogurt or to learn which spices bring out the flavor of lentils. Our food choices need to honor the many worlds we inhabit and connect us to our history, culture, and environment. Fermented foods are a wonderful way to both enrich your diet and connect to the wonders of world cuisine.

CUTTING-EDGE STUDIES:
THE MICROBIOME AND WEIGHT LOSS

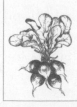

In June 2011 the prestigious *New England Journal of Medicine* reported on research linking yogurt consumption with improved weight. "Intriguing evidence suggests that changes in colonic bacteria might influence weight gain," the article noted. A year earlier the *British Journal of Nutrition* reported that the kinds of bacteria found in yogurt produced improvements in insulin sensitivity and inflammation.

INULIN: A NATURAL PREBIOTIC

Inulin is a type of plant fiber found in the following Microbiome Superfoods:

- Asparagus
- Garlic
- Jerusalem artichoke
- Jicama
- Onion

I also include inulin in your Microbiome Supersupplements.

It's hard to say enough good things about inulin! This plant fiber both nourishes the microbiome and helps heal the gut. It also has terrific weight loss properties.

Inulin decreases the absorption of glucose, a type of sugar, and improves the metabolism of fats. When you consume foods that are rich in inulin, the inulin portion of those foods does not raise your blood sugar levels; in fact, it inhibits your absorption of blood sugar while helping you feel full. Inulin also helps you digest your food more efficiently, which means you'll feel less hungry and, over time, eat less.

Inulin is also crucial for your overall health. When your microbiome gets its daily dose of inulin it is able to produce the vitamins your body requires, particularly vitamins B and K. B vitamins are crucial for coping with stress, managing emotion, thinking clearly, and balancing your hormones. K vitamins are crucial for supporting your metabolism.

Many of us believe we can get our needed quotient of B and K vitamins simply by taking supplements. But the supplements won't do you any good if you don't have a healthy gut—your intestines simply won't be able to absorb them. Many of my patients are shocked when I present them with the results of their vitamin panels. "How can I have a low vitamin B reading?" they ask me. "I take 100 mg a day of a B complex!"

THE SIX KEY BENEFITS OF INULIN

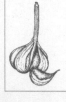

- Feeds healthy bacteria in your microbiome
- Improves digestion
- Inhibits the absorption of glucose so you feel full while absorbing fewer calories
- Supports your body's production of vitamins B and K
- Boosts your metabolism
- Improves bone health

"That supplement won't do you any good if you aren't absorbing it," I reply. That's why supplements aren't enough—we have to heal the gut and rebalance the microbiome. Instead of simply taking supplements, it's far better to eat Microbiome Superfoods rich in inulin so your microbiome will produce its own supply of B and K.

Inulin has also been shown in numerous animal studies to inhibit colon cancer, a finding supported by a 2005 meta-analysis published in the *British Journal of Nutrition*.

Last but not least, inulin helps you absorb calcium and magnesium, which you need to prevent and/or reverse osteoporosis. Again, you can take all the calcium and magnesium supplements you want, but if your gut isn't functioning properly and if you don't have enough inulin in your diet, you won't be able to absorb those expensive pills. The solution? Load up on Microbiome Superfoods so your body has the capacity to absorb the nutrients it needs.

ARABINOGALACTANS: A NATURAL PREBIOTIC

Arabinogalactans is a type of natural prebiotic found in the following Microbiome Superfoods and Microbiome Superspice:

- Carrots
- Onions
- Radishes

- Tomatoes
- Turmeric

Pears, kiwi, and the bark of the larch tree are also rich in arabinogalactans. Pears and kiwi are also featured in the Microbiome Diet. I also include arabinogalactans in your Microbiome Supersupplements.

Arabinogalactans are a plant-based fiber that improves your microbial diversity by feeding the all-important *Lactobacillus*, the type of bacteria used to ferment yogurt and kefir. This natural prebiotic also supports the growth of *Bifidobacterium*, another key type of friendly bacteria.

I like the way arabinogalactans help to combat infections, especially in children. It has strong antibacterial properties, especially against E. coli and a type of unfriendly bacteria known as klebsiella. Overweight people with unhealthy microbiomes often have an overgrowth of klebsiella, which is also associated with autoimmune diseases. Thus, arabinogalactans are terrific for microbial balance, weight loss, and overall immune protection.

In addition, arabinogalactans support natural "killer cell" activity so your immune system can fight off any threats to your body. Even more important, arabinogalactans are natural immune modulators, keeping your immune system in balance. You want an active immune system that attacks any real threat to your system but calms down and relaxes in the face of false threats, such as food products to which you might have become sensitive. An overactive immune system also creates autoimmune conditions, in which your immune system literally begins to attack your own body, including such disorders as Hashimoto's thyroiditis, rheumatoid arthritis, lupus, and multiple sclerosis. Arabinogalactans modulate your immune system and help it walk that middle ground—just active enough, but not overly so. As a result they also have natural anticancer properties.

This type of fiber ferments in your intestinal tract, where it helps fight inflammation and combat allergies. It increases your production of short-chain fatty acids (SCFAs), which, as we saw in earlier

THE SIX KEY BENEFITS OF ARABINOGALACTANS

- Feeds healthy bacteria in your microbiome
- Kills E. coli and klebsiella, which is associated with excess weight and autoimmune conditions
- Supports production of epithelial cells, which strengthen the gut wall
- Anti-inflammatory, which helps combat excess weight
- Overall immune support, which helps prevent auto-immune conditions
- Lowers ammonia levels, which protects your liver

chapters, help support your gut wall as well as protecting your colon from cancer.

Arabinogalactans lower your body's ammonia levels, and this helps support your liver. It also helps prevent cancer elsewhere in your body from metastasizing to your liver.

ASPARAGUS

The beneficial properties of asparagus were noted as early as the second century by the pioneering physician Galen, who noted its ability to cleanse and heal. We've already seen that asparagus is rich in inulin, which feeds the microbiome, thereby leaving you feeling full and helping you lose weight in many different ways.

Asparagus helps to fight inflammation—another aid in the battle to achieve a healthy weight. It helps regulate your blood sugar, which further aids in weight loss.

Asparagus has some anticancer properties. It lowers your body's levels of homocysteine, which could be involved in heart disease and maybe neurological issues. It helps regulate your blood pressure, and it's rich in glutathione, a natural detoxifier, as well as having large quantities of B6, folic acid, vitamin C, beta-carotene, magnesium, chromium, and zinc:

> ## How the Microbiome Superfoods Help You Lose Weight
>
> - Feed your microbiome
> - Balance your blood sugar
> - Leave you feeling full and satisfied
> - Heal your gut walls
> - Fight inflammation
> - Support your digestion through fiber
> - Help rid your body of toxins

- **B6:** supports the body's own production of glutathione and supports the neurotransmitters that keep us energized, optimistic, and focused
- **Folic acid:** supports the body's own production of glutathione
- **Vitamin C:** a key antioxidant that also supports the gut walls
- **Beta-carotene:** a precursor to vitamin A, which is a key antioxidant that also heals the gut wall while supporting vision, cellular health, bone health, and the immune system
- **Magnesium:** needed for digestive enzymes
- **Chromium:** helps move glucose into our cells, combats insulin resistance and thereby promotes fat burning
- **Zinc:** heals gut walls and prevents leaky gut

Tips for Buying and Preparing Asparagus

If you're not used to preparing fresh asparagus, you're in for a treat! This green vegetable always makes me think of springtime, although you can enjoy it any time you can find it in the store.

The key to preparing asparagus well begins at the supermarket. Choose stalks with firm tips so you know you're getting a vegetable that is nice and fresh. Once the asparagus ages, the tips get mushy or furry, which you want to avoid.

You can eat the whole stalk except for the very end—the opposite end from the tip—which you simply cut off. If you've ended up with old asparagus, you might notice that the stalks are woody in texture and white rather than pale green. Cut off those parts—they won't be as good as the tender green stalks.

I like to steam asparagus for about five to eight minutes and then throw on a little lemon and maybe some clarified butter or olive oil. That makes a terrific side dish. You might also steam them and toss them in Lemon Vinaigrette (page 263), and in Phase 2 or 3 you can even add a hard-boiled egg, cut into quarters. That's the traditional French approach to asparagus.

Chef Carole has provided you with a recipe for Roasted Asparagus (page 316). Prepared that way, asparagus has a crispy texture and a nutty, earthy flavor that makes a wonderfully addictive snack.

If you are feeling adventurous, cut up raw stalks of asparagus into small pieces or shave them on a potato grater. Toss them into some mixed greens for a delicious salad and serve with Lemon Vinaigrette (page 263). Raw asparagus tastes very green, crisp, and pungent—a great way to wake up your taste buds.

CARROTS

Carrots have gotten a bad rap for dieters lately because they are high on the glycemic index, meaning they convert to a high level of blood glucose. However, carrots are a fabulous source of arabinogalactans as well as a super source of beta-carotene and vitamin A. As we have seen, vitamin A helps heal the gut walls as well as provide numerous other health benefits.

So carrots appear frequently in the Microbiome Diet, but in small quantities. I'd prefer you not snack on a big bowl of carrots, and you're probably better off not making a salad or side dish entirely out of carrots. But a few carrots among your veggies or in your cooked food adds extraordinary health benefits I don't want you to pass up.

Tips for Buying and Preparing Carrots

I personally prefer to buy carrots that are sold in bunches and *not* in a plastic bag. I think that way they are the freshest and will taste best. Look for firm carrots, not limp, and make sure they have a nice, bright orange color.

You don't have to peel carrots if they're organic; in fact, it's healthier if you don't, because lots of the vitamins and nutrients are in that outer layer of skin. Just scrub them to get the dirt off.

GARLIC

Garlic is one of the most amazing health foods I know. First, it's rich in inulin. It's also loaded with allicin and diallyl sulphides, which support your heart and cardiovascular system in remarkable ways. Among other benefits, garlic is good for:

- Reducing blood pressure
- Lowering cholesterol, both total and LDL (the "bad" cholesterol)
- Lowering oxidative stress
- Reducing the risk of coronary artery disease
- Decreasing the "stickiness" of blood platelets, which helps prevent stroke and other cardiovascular dangers
- Reducing atherosclerotic plaque, also protective against stroke and cardiovascular disease

Garlic responds to our cardiovascular problems so completely that I actually think of it as a wise vegetable that coevolved with us humans almost in mirror image: what we need, it has!

Garlic also increases our body's supply of glutathione, a natural detoxifier, and it reduces the rate of polyps in the colon. Going back to the microbiome, garlic is also good for combating an overgrowth of unfriendly bacteria. With all of these protective effects, no wonder legend has it that garlic also repels vampires!

Tips for Buying and Preparing Garlic

To me, garlic is the king of vegetables: it makes almost every recipe better, and I can't imagine cooking without it. If you're used to using garlic powder, I can't wait for you to switch to the real thing, which has so many more health and flavor benefits that it really is worth the tiny amount of extra trouble involved.

When shopping for fresh garlic you're looking for a moderate-sized white bulb covered in a natural white papery skin. The skin covers many little cloves of garlic, which you will pull away, peel, and chop up. Look for firm bulbs, neither mushy nor dried out.

Please avoid the jars of prechopped garlic—it just doesn't taste the same.

I explain how to cook the garlic in each recipe where I have you use it, but here's my one overall note: you never want to *brown* the garlic, only to warm it up enough to flavor the oil. Cook garlic carefully on a low heat, and you will be rewarded with a delicious subtle taste that wakes up all the other ingredients' flavors.

JERUSALEM ARTICHOKE

If you want to summarize the health benefits of the Jerusalem artichoke in one word, that word would be *inulin*. As we have seen, inulin is a terrific weight loss food that fills you up, balances your blood sugar, and feeds the healthy bacteria in your microbiome. And between 14 and 19 percent of the weight of a Jerusalem artichoke is inulin. Inulin has no calories, but it still leaves you feeling full, making the Jerusalem artichoke one of the best weight loss foods I know. A study by the Center for Health and Nutrition Research at the University of California at Davis found that just six grams of inulin fills you up as completely as 260 calories!

Interestingly, the Jerusalem artichoke is a species of sunflower. So as you are eating the delicious root vegetable, you can picture the large yellow flower, always turning to the sun.

Tips for Buying and Preparing Jerusalem Artichokes

You buy these knobby little vegetables in a one-pound bag. They have a very thin brown skin that can be either peeled or just scrubbed off, exactly the way a potato skin can either be scrubbed or peeled. And like a potato, the skin conceals a starchy snowy-white center, except, unlike the potato, the Jerusalem artichoke "meat" is crispy and sweet.

You can find lots of recipes for Jerusalem artichokes throughout Phase 1 and Phase 2. I grow them in my own garden, so in the fall I also like to serve them raw to my guests. I scrub them well, leaving the skin on, and slice them thin, with a sharp knife or a mandolin (a tool for slicing vegetables, see Pantry List on page 233). Then I dress them with a little virgin olive oil and salt. Mmmm!

You can also steam them, whole or sliced, as a side dish and then dress them with clarified butter and perhaps a squeeze of lemon. Or cut them up into chunks or slices and sauté them in olive oil with some garlic. Throw in some fresh lemon juice, and you have a wonderful sweet and starchy side dish that is just as satisfying and way more healthy than potatoes.

JICAMA

Jicama—pronounced "HICK-uh-muh"—is a root vegetable grown in the Caribbean, Central and South America, and South Asia. If you've ever been to a Mexican restaurant, you've probably noticed it in your salad: a white, crispy, refreshing vegetable with a succulent, fruit-like, sweet-and-starchy taste. It's low in calories (only thirty-five calories per hundred grams) but high in fiber—just what we want to feel full, balance our blood sugar, improve our digestion, and nourish our microbiome.

Besides being high in inulin, jicama has lots of healthy phytonutrients—those plant antioxidants that improve cellular health and fight inflammation. Jicama is also rich in vitamin C, magnesium, and manganese:

- **Vitamin C:** a key antioxidant that also supports the gut walls
- **Magnesium:** needed for digestive enzymes
- **Manganese:** needed for digestive enzymes

These are root vegetables, easily found in the supermarket. Jicama may be in Latin veggies or root vegetable sections.

Tips for Buying and Preparing Jicama

You probably need to look for jicama in the Latin foods section of your grocery store, although you might find it in the produce section. It is a large onion-shaped brown root that has a thick skin, which you'll need to peel. Inside is a sweet, starchy, and succulent white ball that is surprisingly light, crisp, and tangy. You can cut it up into little sticks and munch on it as a snack food, toss it into a salad, or eat it with one of the many dips I suggest in Phases 1 and 2. It's much lighter than a carrot, potato, or parsnip, and if you're serving raw vegetables, jicama is a great addition because its texture is so different from the carrots, celery, and beets that usually go in a raw vegetable dish.

If you are used to snacking on raw carrots, I strongly suggest substituting jicama. You'll get far fewer calories, lots more fiber, and way more support for both weight loss and health.

If you have a family of picky eaters—or if you yourself are cautious about new foods—start small. Throw some in your salad and see how much you enjoy the sweet crunch. You just might find jicama— filling, sweet, and light—one of your favorite snack foods ever.

LEEKS

Leeks are high in both dietary fiber and flavonoids, the antioxidants that support cellular function. They have a lot of manganese, which produces digestive enzymes, as well as high quantities of vitamin A, which is key for healing your gut wall.

Leeks are also high in folate and B6, which supports brain function. Another amazing quality of leeks is their high quantity of kaempferol, which protects us against cancer and cardiovascular disease. It helps us lower blood pressure in two ways: by supporting nitric oxide production and by decreasing our body's production of a compound that blocks nitric oxide production. Leeks also contain polyphenols, which support blood vessel health.

Last but not least, leeks help decrease homocysteine, which can interfere both with your cardiovascular system and with your brain. I like to think about the ways that leeks coevolved with human beings. We humans evolved with certain vulnerabilities in our hearts and our brains, and leeks evolved with us, containing the very nutrients we need to combat those vulnerabilities. This is a good example of drawing upon the intelligence of nature rather than simply relying on the discoveries of science.

Tips for Buying and Preparing Leeks

Leeks look sort of like giant scallions—large green tubes of coiled green skin. They taste very similar to onions, but they have a stronger, greener taste. Look for fresh, green leeks—they should not appear wilted or pale.

The French have always eaten a lot of leeks, but for some reason we Americans don't. If you decide you like leeks, try cutting the leeks into slices, the way you'd slice a scallion or a carrot, and then sautéing them in a little olive oil. Or, if they're not too big, you can simply steam them whole. Then serve warm as a side dish, dressed with butter or oil and some lemon, or serve cold as an appetizer or a salad dressed with Lemon Vinaigrette (page 263).

ONIONS

Onions and garlic come from the same family and share many of the same benefits. Rich in inulin, onions also play a cardioprotective role that is similar to garlic, reducing blood pressure and cholesterol.

They are high in polyphenols, which support our blood vessels. A growing body of research suggests that onions might even play a role in preventing diabetes and cancer.

Onions are also full of flavonoids, antioxidants that improve the integrity of the blood vessels and decrease inflammation. Moreover, they are rich in chromium, which helps regulate our insulin response—another weight loss benefit.

Finally, onions are high in quercitin, which helps heal the gut walls. Although you can find quercitin in supplement form, a recent intriguing study reminds us why it's important to eat foods and not simply consume supplements. In the study some animals were fed yellow onion while others were just given quercitin. The animals that ate the actual food enjoyed the greatest health benefits.

Tips for Buying and Preparing Onions

You're probably quite familiar with the onion, so I'll just throw out a couple of suggestions. First, look for onions that are firm, not mushy, and try to avoid onions that have sprouted. Second, when you are making soup stock you can wash the onion well without peeling it and include the onion skin in the soup for some extra color.

RADISHES

Radishes have won their status as a Microbiome Superfood because of their high amount of arabinogalactans. They are a wonderful snack food—filling, nutritious, and nourishing to your microbiome. Radishes are also high in magnesium and manganese (crucial for the production of digestive enzymes), vitamin C (a terrific antioxidant and immune system support), calcium (for bone health), folate, and vitamin B6 (good for coping with stress and supporting brain function). To make matters even better, they have a mild anti-inflammatory effect, which, as we know, helps to combat weight gain.

Tips for Buying and Preparing Radishes

I love radishes! They add a spicy crunch to a salad, and I also like to eat them plain with dip. There are many varieties of radish available, but the most common are the small red bulbs with the green leaves on top. Scrub the skin but don't peel it. If you slice a radish, it's white inside, but the red skin adds a nice bit of color, so don't scrub it off.

If you're putting radishes into a salad or smoothie, cut off the greens. But I like to leave the greens on and put them out for guests with a bowl of extra-virgin olive oil and a little bowl of sea salt. Dip them in the oil first, then the salt, and enjoy! Or slice the radishes in half lengthwise (without the greens) and spread a very thin layer of butter and some salt—very French! When you get into Phases 2 and 3 of the Microbiome Diet you can also spread a little chèvre or goat cheese onto a half radish for a quick and delicious snack.

TOMATOES

This Microbiome Superfood is rich in arabinogalactans, one of the types of dietary fiber that nourishes your microbiome while supporting your digestion and leaving you feeling full. Its bright red color indicates it is full of lycopene, an outstanding antioxidant, and the vitamin C in tomatoes adds to its antioxidant protection.

Tomatoes are also rich in vitamin A, which, as we have seen, is an important gut-healing vitamin in addition to all its other benefits. Tomatoes lower cholesterol and triglycerides and reduce platelet stickiness, giving them great cardioprotective benefits.

Last but not least, tomatoes are also good for bone health, so they are a terrific addition to your diet if you are at risk for osteoporosis.

Tips for Buying and Preparing Tomatoes

I personally never buy tomatoes out of season—I use canned tomatoes instead. Look for canned organic tomatoes if possible. My personal approach to buying tomatoes is to smell them—if it doesn't smell like a tomato, it won't taste like one. Look for tomatoes that are bright tomato red, firm but not mushy or woody. When you prepare them don't peel them; just wash them gently and cut them up. Cut away any mealy, green, or woody portions.

HEALTHY FATS TO FOCUS ON

As we have seen, healthy fats are crucial for cell health and healing the intestinal walls. In the Microbiome Diet we load you up with the healthiest possible fats:

- Nuts and nut butters—almond, macadamia
- Seeds and seed butters—sunflower seed butter
- Flaxseed and flaxseed oil
- Sunflower seed oil
- Olive oil

You also get healthy fish oil in the fish dishes on your meal plans.

You don't need to obsess about the balance of Omega 3s and Omega 6s. Just make sure you are focusing on healthy fats and have some fish, flax, nuts, or seeds each day. Following the Phase 1 and Phase 2 meal plans will accustom you to naturally balancing your fats.

WHAT ABOUT VEGETARIANS AND VEGANS?

There are several vegetarian dishes on the Microbiome Diet but probably not enough to sustain a seven-week diet. It can be very difficult to lose weight as a vegetarian or vegan, especially when you are trying to avoid gluten, dairy, soy, and eggs in support of digestive health.

If you are committed to eating as a vegetarian or vegan, I suggest you focus on adding the Microbiome Superfoods, Superspices, and Supersupplements to your diet and work with a nutritionist to make sure you are getting enough protein and other nutrients.

MAKE THE HEALTHIEST CHOICES

The benefits of eating organic, free-range, and cruelty-free food are well documented. I realize these choices are often more expensive than conventionally farmed or industrially produced food, but in the long run you will save more money eating this way.

First, in the long run you will eat less. As your microbiome and your intestinal tract are freed of the chemicals added to conventionally produced food, including antibiotics and the stress chemicals from the bodies of badly treated animals, your hunger will adjust to what your body really needs. You may be surprised at the extent to which the Microbiome Diet affects your appetite.

Second, by not using processed, packaged foods you save money as well. Premade foods often cost more than organic, whole-food alternatives.

Finally, your improved health will save you money on doctor's bills, missed days of work, and over-the-counter remedies for the colds, coughs, sleep problems, headaches, and other ailments you will no longer experience once your gut is in good shape and your microbiome is rebalanced. So please, if you can, choose as follows:

- Organic fruits and vegetables
- Wild-caught salmon and unfarmed fish
- Meat, eggs, and dairy from free-range, grass-fed animals that have been treated as humanely as possible

MICROBIOME SWEET TREATS

You'll notice that I've asked you to avoid all sugars and sweeteners, natural or artificial, except for a product called Lakanto. Sugar and natural sweeteners (honey, maple syrup, agave) feed unhealthy bacteria and unbalance your microbiome. Artificial sweeteners harm your microbiome also. And both types of sweeteners stress your liver in different ways. Many diet book authors recommend stevia and/or

continues

continued

MICROBIOME SWEET TREATS

xylitol as natural substances that are also healthy sweeteners. Although these alternatives are certainly preferable to either sugar or artificial sweeteners, Lakanto is your healthiest choice. Made from a fermented sugar alcohol known as erythritol and from an extract of the Chinese *luo han guo* fruit, Lakanto helps to create the short-chain fatty acids (SC-FAs) that are so beneficial to your health and weight.

You'll also notice that on the Microbiome Diet we have no recipes for desserts, nor do the meal plans include desserts. When you get to the 90 percent compliance of Phase 2 and the 70 percent compliance of Phase 3 you can add in a few desserts if you like. But I'd rather you train your palate to appreciate the Microbiome Superfoods and Superspices, focusing on the delicious tastes of nutritious foods rather than thinking of dessert as the "treat." The Microbiome Diet will leave you feeling full and satisfied, so try eating without desserts for a while.

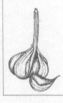

Of course, there are plenty of sweet treats on the Microbiome Diet—mango smoothies, granola, fruit compote, and many others. But I'd love you to incorporate your sweetness into a meal rather than thinking of it as the reward for finishing. Give yourself a few weeks to find out whether you start to appreciate other foods more so the meal itself becomes the treat.

twelve

PHASE 1:
YOUR FOUR Rs MEAL PLAN

IN PHASE 1 OF THE MICROBIOME DIET YOU WILL IMPLEMENT THE Four Rs of intestinal health. The foods and supplements for this phase of the diet have been chosen with the following goals in mind:

- **Remove** the unhealthy bacteria and the foods that unbalance the microbiome.
- **Replace** the stomach acid and digestive enzymes you need for optimal digestion.
- **Reinoculate** with probiotics (intestinal bacteria) and prebiotics (substances that nourish this bacteria and keep it healthy).
- **Repair** the lining of your intestinal walls, which have likely become permeable and are releasing partially digested food into your bloodstream, with disastrous results.

I tell my patients that a healthy body regulates its own weight so you feel hungry when you really need food and full when you have eaten all you require. A healthy body also craves the foods it needs, with little interest in the foods that do not support it.

So if you weigh more than your ideal weight, by definition, your microbiome is out of balance and your gut is in distress. Likewise, if you feel hungry most of the time or if you frequently crave sugar, starches, or dairy, your system is out of balance.

Follow the Four Rs Meal Plan, and in twenty-one days you will feel like a different person. Your weight will begin to come off. Your skin and hair will glow. You will feel calmer, more energized, sharper, and more focused. You will feel free of the hunger and the cravings that now seem to hold you prisoner. And thanks to Chef Carole Clark's wonderful meals, you will have eaten in a way that satisfies your senses and makes every mealtime a treat.

Here's something else I tell my patients: Eat until you are only about 80 percent full. If you are overweight, your body has probably gotten used to consuming more food than you need, so your signals for "hunger" and "fullness" are somewhat out of balance. Eat to that 80 percent mark—in my experience, that ends up being a meal about one-half the size that you are used to—and see how your feelings of hunger and fullness shift.

FOODS TO REMOVE

The following are the foods we are removing in the Four Rs phase of the Microbiome Diet. After twenty-one days, when your gut is healed and your microbiome is beginning to come into balance, we can add a few of these foods back in.

For these twenty-one days, however, I would like you to follow the meal plans and restrictions very closely. Think of this diet as a medical prescription that is helping your system to heal. Please avoid all of the following foods:

- Processed or packaged foods

- High-fructose corn syrup
- Trans fats
- Hydrogenated fats
- Dried or canned fruits
- Juices
- Gluten
- All grains, including rice and quinoa
- Corn and cornstarch
- All sugars and sweeteners, natural or artificial, except Lakanto
- All dairy products—milk, yogurt, cheese—except butter and ghee (clarified butter)
- Eggs
- Soy, including soy milk, soy sauce, tofu, tempeh, and all forms of soy isolate protein such as are found in many protein bars, protein shakes, and protein powders (check the label!), except soy lecithin
- Processed meats or deli meats
- Peanuts or peanut butter
- Canola oil or cottonseed oil
- Potatoes, sweet potatoes, or yams
- Legumes: black, white, red, or kidney beans; fava beans; and string beans (yes, these are legumes), except chickpeas/garbanzo beans and lentils
- Iceberg lettuce

Here is how avoiding these foods will benefit your microbiome and your entire intestinal system:

Processed or packaged foods. These contain so many ingredients that stress your gut and imbalance your microbiome that it's hard to know where to start! Preservatives and food coloring stress your liver and make it harder for that vital organ to metabolize fat, and this can lead to weight gain. Packaged foods often contain gluten as a preservative. As we saw in Chapter 3, gluten produces zonulin, which causes the tight junctions in your intestinal walls to open, leading to leaky gut, immune reactions, inflammation, and weight gain. Packaged foods also often contain soy, which can trigger immune reactions if you have leaky gut and is almost certainly genetically modified, posing dangers to your microbiome. Packaged foods usually include trans fats, hydrogenated fats, and/or canola oil, each of which threatens your microbiome and your health in numerous ways (see below). Finally, packaged foods often contain high-fructose corn syrup, which creates so many problems that I could write an entire book on that alone!

High-fructose corn syrup. This sweetener feeds unhealthy bacteria. Because most of the corn in the United States has been genetically modified, HFCS also scrambles your "second genome." Because of the way fructose is metabolized in your body, HFCS stresses your liver, disrupting your body's ability to get rid of toxins and metabolize fat. I really can't say enough bad things about high-fructose corn syrup and neither can any physician, nutritionist, or health professional I know. If you want to rebalance your microbiome, heal your gut, and lose weight, avoid this substance, please!

Trans and hydrogenated fats. These are the unhealthy fats found in processed foods, the ones that lead to immediate inflammation. Trans and hydrogenated fats have been modified to give them a longer shelf life, but as a result they don't support your cells the way healthy fats do. Healthy fats are a key component of the Microbiome Diet because they are crucial to cell creation and repair, making them vital for both gut health and optimal brain function. Focus on healthy fats while avoiding trans and hydrogenated fats at all costs. They imbalance your microbiome, create inflammation, and lead to almost instant weight gain.

Dried or canned fruits. These seemingly healthy foods often contain added sugar and therefore imbalance your microbiome: they feed glucose and fructose to the unhealthy bacteria. They also set up a craving for sweets by feeding yeast and other sugar-loving microbes.

Juices. When you juice a food you take out the fiber, and as we have seen, the fiber is what feeds the microbiome. Fruit juices are too high in fructose, which feeds your unhealthy bacteria, although when you get to Your Lifetime Tune-Up, vegetable juices might be a healthy choice. At this point in your healing process, however, stick to whole fruits and vegetables only. Even the seemingly healthy fresh juices you buy as they are prepared in front of you are often loaded with apple juice, and the packaged "healthy" juices are definitely full of fruit juices, even the ones that call themselves "green" (check the ingredients list if you don't believe me). Whole foods—not juiced ones—are your best choices for now.

Gluten. Gluten creates zonulin, which opens the tight junctions in your intestinal wall and helps create leaky gut.

All grains, including rice. Gluten-free grains such as rice, millet, and quinoa can be healthy choices, and we include them in the next phase of the Microbiome Diet. For this first cleansing phase, however, I'd like you to avoid them because they do support some unhealthy bacteria, including yeast. Rice and millet also contain lectins, a substance that blocks mineral absorption, so they should always be eaten in moderation. However, when your microbiome is better balanced you will be able to enjoy some gluten-free grains.

Corn and cornstarch. Most US corn is genetically modified, making it dangerous both to your microbiome and to your entire system. Corn is a sweet, starchy grain, so it can feed your unhealthy bacteria while your microbiome is still unbalanced.

All sugars and sweeteners, natural or artificial, except Lakanto. As we have seen, sugar and natural sweeteners feed unhealthy bacteria and unbalance your microbiome, as do artificial sweeteners. Moreover, both natural and artificial sweeteners stress your liver. I recommend that if you are looking for a sugar substitute, focus on Lakanto (see page 64). Although stevia and xylitol are natural substances and preferable to either sugar or artificial sweeteners, I urge you to stick to Lakanto.

All dairy products—milk, yogurt, cheese—except butter and ghee (clarified butter). Dairy products are healthful for many people, and unless you are lactose intolerant or have an ongoing intolerance for dairy, you will be able to add these products back into your diet in Phase 2, the Metabolic Boost. But while you have leaky gut—and if you are overweight, you almost by definition have it—you need to avoid foods that can cause your immune system to react. Because dairy products are among the most reactive foods, I'm suggesting you cut them out during this healing phase. Because butter and ghee contain only fat—no milk protein—they are safe in this phase.

Eggs. Eggs, both the whites and the yolks, are among the most healthful foods on earth, but if you have leaky gut, you may be reactive to eggs as well. I've saved them for the next phase of the Microbiome Diet, when your healthy gut and improved microbiome can tolerate them. I suspect that much of the problem with eggs represents a reaction to the corn, soy, and other unhealthy feed given to the industrially raised chickens that lay them. When you do eat eggs, buy organic, free-range eggs whenever you possibly can.

Soy, including soy milk, soy sauce, tofu, tempeh, miso, and all forms of soy isolate protein such as are found in many protein bars, protein shakes, and protein powders (check the label!), except soy lecithin. Besides being genetically modified, soy is another potentially reactive food for many people with leaky gut. Soy also poses grave problems for women because of the ways it affects estrogen production. Soy is challenging to the thyroid as well. In any case, the only form of soy that is healthy for humans is fermented soy, as is found in miso and tofu; soy isolate protein is very difficult for humans to digest. Although the soy industry did a great advertising job promoting soy as a healthy food, I believe just the opposite is true. Although I know many well-respected people who would disagree with me, I believe soy poses numerous risks to your health, and genetically modified soy creates even greater risks. You would do best to avoid it.

Processed meats or deli meats. These are likely to be loaded with gluten not to mention trans or hydrogenated fats. Stay away from them.

Peanuts or peanut butter. Peanuts are not nuts, they are legumes, and as such they contain lectins, which interfere with mineral absorption. They also often contain aflotoxin, a toxin found in various molds, which is dangerous to your microbial balance.

Canola oil or cottonseed oil. Canola oil is actually rapeseed oil, an industrial oil that was not originally intended for cooking. The rapeseed has been genetically modified, creating the dangers to your "second genome." There is also evidence that over time canola oil destroys the myelin sheath that coats your nerves, creating numerous disturbing symptoms.

Potatoes, sweet potatoes, or yams. These can be healthy foods in moderation, especially sweet potatoes and yams. However, they are high in starch, which can feed unhealthy bacteria. Enjoy these foods in Phase 3, when your microbiome is more balanced.

Legumes: black, white, red, or kidney beans; fava beans; string beans, except chickpeas/garbanzo beans and lentils. Legumes can be wonderful sources of protein, fiber, vitamins, and minerals, but while you have leaky gut they are hard for your intestinal tract to handle. They also contain lectins, which interfere with mineral absorption. Chickpeas and lentils are easier to digest and have so many nutritional benefits that I am including them even in Phase 1. These foods include *raffinose* and *stachyose*, which are highly beneficial to your microbiome, as well as *resistant starches,* a type of fiber that is a powerful prebiotic.

Iceberg lettuce. This is the least nutritious of all the lettuces and is loaded with toxic insecticides that can disrupt your microbiome. Avoid it in favor of dark green lettuce, which is far healthier.

YOUR MICROBIOME SUPERFOODS

As we saw in the previous section, there are some Superfoods and Superspices that are heavily featured throughout the Microbiome Diet:

Natural probiotics, which replenish your microbiome with more healthy bacteria:

- Fermented foods, especially sauerkraut, kimchee, and kefir and yogurt made from sheep's or goat's milk

Natural prebiotics, which nourish the healthy bacteria already in your microbiome:

- Asparagus
- Carrots
- Garlic
- Jerusalem artichoke
- Jicama
- Leeks
- Onions
- Radishes
- Tomatoes

Superspices:

- Cinnamon, which balances blood sugar and, therefore, insulin, working against insulin resistance and cuing your body to burn fat rather than store it
- Turmeric, a natural anti-inflammatory, that helps heal the gut, support the microbiome, and promote good brain function as well as having anticancer properties

HEALTHY FOODS

These are healthy foods you can enjoy throughout all phases of the Microbiome Diet. Note that all nuts should be eaten raw, never roasted, as that destroys many of their healthy properties.

Proteins	
beef	lamb
chicken	shellfish
fish (low-mercury only)	

Vegetables	
artichoke	cucumber
asparagus	eggplant
beets	garlic
berries	kale
black radish	kohlrabi
bok choy	lettuce—anything but iceberg
broccoli and broccolini, broccoli rabe	mushrooms
brussels sprouts	onions
cabbages	spinach
capers	squash
carrots (in cooking, not as a snack or side dish)	tomatoes
	turnips
cauliflower	watercress
celery	zucchini

Fruits	
apples (no more than one a day)	grapefruit
avocado	kiwi
cherries	nectarines
coconut	orange
coconut water	rhubarb

Nuts and Seeds	
almonds	nut flours
Brazil nuts	walnuts

Oils	
butter or ghee (organic); ghee is better	coconut milk (unsweetened)
coconut oil	

Legumes	
chick peas (garbanzos)	lentils

PORTION SIZES

With a few exceptions I have not included portion sizes in the Microbiome Diet. This diet is not about counting calories or measuring out portions—it is about healing your gut, rebalancing your microbiome, and restoring your natural sense of hunger and full-ness. If you stick to the foods on the meal plan and follow portion sizes when I do give them, you are unlikely to go very far wrong. Focus on pleasure, not measure!

PHASE 1 YOUR FOUR Rs MEAL PLAN:
TWENTY-ONE DAYS TO GUT INTEGRITY

Here are twenty-one days' worth of meal plans. The asterisk denotes recipes provided.

These three delicious meals and two snacks are designed to leave you feeling satisfied in every way. I have you eating fermented foods because, as we have seen, they contain live cultures that replenish your microbiome. You can choose which types of fermented food you prefer—kimchee, sauerkraut, or fermented vegetables of any type. Make sure the fermented foods you buy are made without whey, which is a form of dairy, and of course, choose organic products. In the Resources I have suggested sources for buying high-quality fermented foods online, or you can find them at your grocery store. Because you might not be used to eating fermented foods, I have you work your way up gradually from small to larger amounts.

Even though the Microbiome Diet has everything you need, you might find yourself feeling hungry after a meal or between meals as you make the transition to this new way of eating. If so, my suggestion is that you load up on kimchee, raw sauerkraut, or fermented vegetables, all of which are both filling and very supportive of your microbiome. You can also add any of the choices below to any of your meals or snacks:

- Salad with Lemon Vinaigrette* and any of the following ingredients: lettuce (except iceberg), watercress, asparagus, cucumber, red peppers, red or green onion. Including half an avocado will add a few more healthy fats.

- Broccoli, broccolini, kale, collards, kohlrabi.
- The following snacks from the meal plan: Curried Roasted Cauliflower*, Oven-Roasted Kale Chips*, sliced Jerusalem artichoke, Roasted Asparagus with Lemon*.

*DENOTES RECIPES PROVIDED

I'd like you to basically avoid alcohol in Phases 1 and 2 because of its potentially stressful impact on the microbiome. In Phase 3 you can include some alcoholic beverages as part of your 30 percent indulgence. In all three phases I advise limiting your caffeinated coffee intake to one or two eight-ounce cups per day, and your caffeinated tea intake to three to five eight-ounce cups per day. You can have as much decaf coffee and herbal tea as you like. Please avoid fruit juices, which are the least healthy way to consume fruit—you really want the fiber along with the fructose! Vegetable juices can be healthy if they are fresh and really contain only veggies, but watch out for the commercially bottled ones, which usually have a high quantity of fruit juice. They may be "natural," as their labels proclaim, but they are not necessarily healthy, especially if you are trying to lose weight.

YOUR MICROBIOME SUPERSUPPLEMENTS

Take these supplements any time of day you like, with or without meals, unless otherwise specified.

To remove unhealthy bacteria from your intestines, you have two choices:

1) You can look for a combination product that contains the following ingredients:

   - Berberine
   - Wormwood
   - Caprylic acid
   - Grapefruit seed extract

- Garlic
- Oregano Oil

I have recommended a few good combination products in the Resources section. Just follow the directions on the bottle for dosage.

2) You can take a single product. Choose either:

- Garlic, 5000 micrograms, three times a day

OR

- Berberine, 200 mg, three times a day

To Replace Stomach Acid

- Hydrochloric acid, 1000 mg with each meal

OR

- Apple cider vinegar, 1 teaspoon diluted with 5 to 6 tea-spoons of water, with each meal. Gradually increase the dose until you are drinking 3 to 4 teaspoons of vinegar with each meal.

To Replace Enzymes

Find a good combination product that includes:

- Protease, which digests protein
- Lipase, which digests fat
- Amylase, which digests starches
- DPP 41V, which helps digest gluten and casein (milk protein) in case trace elements end up in your meal

Take one to two pills per meal. I have recommended some good combination products in Resources.

REINOCULATE WITH PROBIOTICS

1. Find a good probiotic with the following qualities:

- The more diverse species, the better
- Should contain at least these three types of *Lactobacillus*: *acidophilous, rameneses, planataris*
- Should contain different types of *Bifidobacter*
- A bonus if it contains *Acidophilus reuterii*
- Should contain between 50 billion and 200 billion bacteria—the more, the better

Take one pill or packet a day. I have recommended some good brands in Resources.

2. For weight loss take *Acidophilus gasseri*, which you will have to buy separately unless you have purchased one of the few probiotics that contains it. I have recommended some sources in Resources. Take as directed.

REINOCULATE WITH PREBIOTICS

1. Take inulin powder: 4 to 6 grams a day, divided into two doses
2. Take arabinogalactans, 500 to 1000 mg, two times a day

You can also look for a combination of inulin and arabinogala-catans. I have recommended some good combination products in Resources.

3. Take cal-mag butyrate, 200 to 300 mg, one to two times a day. Butyrate is both a prebiotic and a weight loss supplement.

REPAIR WITH SUPPLEMENTS

When you look for supplements to repair the gut, you'd do best to find a combination product, either in pill or powder form—I prefer powder. Some of the individual ingredients to look for include the following (or you can take them individually in the doses listed):

1. Glutamine: 1 to 5 grams a day
2. Quercitin: 100 to 500 mg a day; look for "iso-quercitin," which is better absorbed
3. Zinc alone or with carnosine. If in combination, 100 to 150 mg a day. If you take zinc by itself, take 30 mg a day, and then take carnosine in a dose of 100 to 500 mg a day.
4. N-acetyl glucosamine, 1000 mg a day
5. DGL (diglycerinated licorice), 400 mg a day
6. Slippery Elm, 200 mg a day
7. Marshmallow, 100 mg a day
8. Gamma Oryzanol, 300 mg to 1.5 grams a day

You can also take a combination product. I recommend several in Resources.

ADDITIONAL WEIGHT LOSS AIDS

1. Meratrim: 400 mg, two times a day, thirty minutes before breakfast and dinner.
2. *Sphaeranthus indicus* and *Garcinia mangostana*. You can buy them separately and follow the directions on the bottle, or look for a formula that includes those compounds and meratrim. Some combinations include capsicum, which offers additional weight loss benefits, as well as zychrome, which helps to balance blood sugar. See Resources for some suggestions.
3. Green coffee bean extract, 400 mg, two times a day
   OR
   Irvingia (African mango), 150 to 300 mg, two times a day

MEAL PLANS FOR THE MICROBIOME DIET

PHASE ONE

WEEK 1

DAY 1

BREAKFAST
Sunrise Smoothie*

SNACK
Jicama and radish slices with sunflower seed butter

LUNCH
Prebiotic Superfood Green Salad with Lemon Vinaigrette*

SNACK
Raspberries and blueberries with ten almonds

DINNER
Lemon Chicken Stew*, 2 tablespoons kimchee

DAY 2

BREAKFAST
Minted Fruit Salad with Brazil Nuts*

SNACK
Celery and parsnip sticks with almond butter

LUNCH
Traditional Chicken Soup*

SNACK
Curried Roasted Cauliflower*

DINNER
Pan-Roasted Salmon* on Fennel Salad* with
Lemon Vinaigrette,* watercress, and mixed greens,
2½ tablespoons fermented beets or your choice of
fermented vegetables

MEAL PLANS FOR THE MICROBIOME DIET

DAY 3

BREAKFAST
Half grapefruit and orange sections with cinnamon and strawberries

SNACK
Cherry tomatoes and Jerusalem artichoke slices with sunflower seed butter

LUNCH
Guacamole Smoothie*

SNACK
Curried Roasted Cauliflower* (use leftovers from Day 2)

DINNER
Beef, Beer, and Onion Stew*, 3 tablespoons your choice of fermented vegetables

DAY 4

BREAKFAST
Sunrise Smoothie*

SNACK
Tomato, Jerusalem artichoke slices, cucumber, and radish with olive oil and sea salt dips

LUNCH
Sauerkraut and Meatball Soup*

SNACK
Oven-Roasted Kale Chips*

DINNER
Lemon Chicken Stew* (use leftovers from Day 1), 3½ tablespoons your choice of fermented vegetables

MEAL PLANS FOR THE MICROBIOME DIET

DAY 5

BREAKFAST
Mango Smoothie*

SNACK
Curried Roasted Cauliflower* (use leftovers from Day 2) and ten cashews

LUNCH
Asparagus Salad with Lemon Vinaigrette*

SNACK
Kiwi and berries

DINNER
Beef, Beer, and Onion Stew* (use leftovers from Day 3), 4 tablespoons your choice of fermented vegetables

DAY 6

BREAKFAST
Nectarine Kiwi Smoothie*

SNACK
Steamed Artichoke with Lemon Mustard Dip*

LUNCH
Chicken Salad with Fennel, Tomato, Olives, Jicama, and Greens*

SNACK
Oven-Roasted Kale Chips*

DINNER
Meatballs with Roasted Spaghetti Squash and Basil Pesto*, 4½ tablespoons your choice of fermented vegetables

MEAL PLANS FOR THE MICROBIOME DIET

WEEK 2

DAY 7

BREAKFAST
Minted Fruit Salad with Brazil Nuts*

SNACK
Carrot and celery sticks with sunflower seed butter

LUNCH
Traditional Chicken Soup* (use the soup you made and froze on Day 2)

SNACK
Spiced Roasted Chickpeas*

DINNER
Seared Scallops* with Easy Sautéed Greens*, 5 tablespoons your choice of fermented vegetables

DAY 8

BREAKFAST
Half grapefruit with cinnamon and berries and ten walnuts

SNACK
Oven-Roasted Kale Chips*

LUNCH
Gazpacho Smoothie*

SNACK
Steamed Artichoke with Lemon Mustard Dip* (use leftover dip from Day 6)

DINNER
Curried Lamb and Lentil Stew*, mixed green salad, 5½ tablespoons your choice of fermented vegetables

MEAL PLANS FOR THE MICROBIOME DIET

DAY 9

BREAKFAST
Mango Smoothie*

SNACK
Roasted Asparagus with Lemon* with ten almonds

LUNCH
Rich Vegetable Soup*

SNACK
Spiced Roasted Chickpeas* (use leftover Spiced Roasted Chickpeas from Day 7; to make them crisp, reheat in 350°F oven until hot)

DINNER
Curried Lamb and Lentil Stew* (use leftovers from Day 8), 6 tablespoons your choice of fermented vegetables

DAY 10

BREAKFAST
Minted Fruit Salad with Brazil Nuts*

SNACK
Guacamole Smoothie*

LUNCH
Rumanian Eggplant Salad*

SNACK
Oven-Roasted Kale Chips*

DINNER
Beef Stew with Aromatic Vegetables and Red Wine*, 6 tablespoons your choice of fermented vegetables

MEAL PLANS FOR THE MICROBIOME DIET

DAY 11

BREAKFAST
Sunrise Smoothie*

SNACK
Spiced Roasted Chickpeas*

LUNCH
Chicken Soup with Kale and Jerusalem Artichokes*
(use frozen Chicken Base prepared at the beginning
of the diet)

SNACK
Roasted Asparagus with Lemon* and almonds (use
leftover roasted asparagus from the Asparagus Salad*
you made on Day 5)

DAY 12

BREAKFAST
Orange and grapefruit sections with cinnamon

SNACK
Medley of raw vegetables with Basil Pesto*

LUNCH
Sauerkraut and Meatball Soup* (use the extra serving
you froze on Day 4)

SNACK
Nuts and berries

DINNER
Braised Apple Chicken* with mixed green salad,
6 tablespoons your choice of fermented vegetables

MEAL PLANS FOR THE MICROBIOME DIET

DAY 13

BREAKFAST
Citrusy Avocado Compote*

SNACK
Gazpacho Smoothie*

LUNCH
Stuffed Mushrooms* on Easy Sautéed Greens*
(try broccoli rabe)

SNACK
Jerusalem artichoke slices and cherry tomatoes with
olive oil and sea salt dips

DINNER
Fish Stew with Romesco*, mixed green salad,
6 tablespoons your choice of fermented vegetable

DAY 14

BREAKFAST
Nectarine Kiwi Smoothie*

SNACK
Apple slices with almond butter

LUNCH
Arugula Salad*

SNACK
Steamed Artichoke with Lemon Mustard Dip* (use the
extra dip from Day 6)

DINNER
Curried Vegetable Stew*, 6 tablespoons your choice of
fermented vegetables

MEAL PLANS FOR THE MICROBIOME DIET

WEEK 3

DAY 15

BREAKFAST
Minted Fruit Salad with Brazil Nuts*

SNACK
Spiced Roasted Chickpeas* (use leftover Spiced Roasted Chickpeas* from Day 7; to make them crisp, put in 350°F oven until hot)

LUNCH
Rumanian Eggplant Salad* (use the leftover Rumanian Eggplant Salad from Day 10)

SNACK
Guacamole Smoothie*

DINNER
Meatballs with Roasted Spaghetti Squash and Basil Pesto* (use leftover Meatballs and Roasted Spaghetti Squash from Day 6), 6 tablespoons your choice of fermented vegetables

DAY 16

BREAKFAST
Sunrise Smoothie*

SNACK
Carrot, jicama, and celery sticks with Basil Pesto* (use the extra Basil Pesto* from Day 6)

LUNCH
Traditional Chicken Soup* (use the Chicken Stock you made at the beginning of the diet)

SNACK
Stuffed Mushrooms* (use leftover Stuffed Mushrooms from Day 13)

DINNER
Seared Scallops* with Easy Sautéed Greens* (try Swiss chard), 6 tablespoons your choice of fermented vegetables

MEAL PLANS FOR THE MICROBIOME DIET

DAY 17

BREAKFAST
Grapefruit and orange sections with cinnamon

SNACK
Oven-Roasted Kale Chips*

LUNCH
Green salad with fennel, tomato, asparagus, Jerusalem artichoke, radish with Lemon Vinaigrette*

SNACK
Apple slices with almond butter

DINNER
Curried Lamb and Lentil Stew* (use leftover frozen Curried Lamb and Lentil Stew* from Day 9), 6 tablespoons your choice of fermented vegetables

DAY 18

BREAKFAST
Minted Fruit Salad with Brazil Nuts*

SNACK
Cherry tomatoes, jicama, red peppers, and cucumbers with Romesco* used as a dip (use the extra Romesco* from Day 13)

LUNCH
Rumanian Eggplant Salad* (use leftover Rumanian Eggplant Salad from Day 10)

SNACK
Oven-Roasted Kale Chips*

DINNER
Pan-Roasted Salmon* on Fennel Salad* with Lemon Vinaigrette*, watercress, and mixed greens, 6 tablespoons your choice of fermented vegetables

MEAL PLANS FOR THE MICROBIOME DIET

DAY 19

BREAKFAST
Nectarine Kiwi Smoothie*

SNACK
Roasted Asparagus with Lemon* with ten almonds

LUNCH
Arugula Salad*

SNACK
Spiced Roasted Chickpeas*

DINNER
Curried Vegetable Stew* (use leftover Curried Vegetable Stew from Day 14), 6 tablespoons your choice of fermented vegetables

DAY 20

BREAKFAST
Mango Smoothie*

SNACK
Steamed Artichoke with Lemon Mustard Dip* (use the extra Lemon Mustard Dip* from Day 6)

LUNCH
Sauerkraut and Meatball Soup* (use frozen Sauerkraut and Meatball Soup from Day 4)

SNACK
Roasted Asparagus with Lemon* with ten almonds (use leftover Roasted Asparagus from Day 19)

DINNER
Braised Apple Chicken* (use frozen Braised Apple Chicken from Day 12) with mixed green salad, 6 tablespoons your choice of fermented vegetable

MEAL PLANS FOR THE MICROBIOME DIET

DAY 21

BREAKFAST

Half grapefruit with berries and cinnamon, four Brazil nuts

SNACK

Spiced Roasted Chickpeas* (use leftover Spiced Roasted Chickpeas from Day 19)

LUNCH

Chicken Soup with Kale and Jerusalem Artichokes* (use the frozen Chicken Base you made at the beginning of the diet)

SNACK

Apple slices with almond butter

DINNER

Beef Stew with Aromatic Vegetables and Red Wine* (use leftover Beef Stew you froze on Day 10), 6 tablespoons your choice of fermented vegetables

thirteen

PHASE 2: YOUR METABOLIC BOOST MEAL PLAN

CONGRATULATIONS! NOW YOU HAVE COMPLETED THE FIRST TWENTY-ONE days of the Microbiome Diet. Your leaky gut is well on its way to healing, perhaps even completely healed. Your microbiome is in much better shape, but there is still more work to do. So in this phase of the Microbiome Diet you will completely avoid all foods that do serious damage to your Microbiome Diet while continuing to load up on healing and fermented foods.

PRINCIPLES OF THE METABOLIC BOOST MEAL PLAN

Our goal in the next four weeks is to give you a real metabolic boost. Improving the health of your microbiome helps reduce your body's inflammatory burden. This in turn cues your insulin response to switch from fat storage to fat burning.

Altering your approach to every meal will help as well, as you switch from stressed-out eating to stress-free eating. Pausing before you eat so you can switch from the "fight or flight" stress response to the "rest and digest" relaxation response—from the sympathetic to the parasympathetic nervous systems—will give you an enormous metabolic boost. So during the next four weeks I want you to practice stress-free eating. The delicious foods Chef Carole Clark has planned for you will help you savor your food and enjoy your meals and snack times to the fullest.

90 PERCENT COMPLIANCE

Because your intestinal tract and your microbiome are so much stronger, you have a bit more leeway on this phase of the Microbiome Diet. You are free to maintain only 90 percent compliance. That means that of the thirty-five meals and snacks you consume during a week, three or four of them can include a food that is not included on the meal plan or in my list of acceptable foods. However, there are still some foods you should make sure to avoid.

FOODS TO AVOID

As I explained in Phase 1, the following foods are so unhealthy for your intestinal tract and your microbiome that you need to avoid them throughout Phase 2 as well. Please avoid all of the following foods:

- Processed or packaged foods
- High-fructose corn syrup
- Trans fats
- Hydrogenated fats
- Dried or canned fruits
- Juices
- Gluten

- Soy, including soy milk, soy sauce, tofu, tempeh, and all forms of soy isolate protein such as are found in many protein bars, protein shakes, and protein powders (check the label!), except soy lecithin
- Processed meats or deli meats
- Peanuts or peanut butter
- Canola oil or cottonseed oil

FOODS TO ADD BACK IN

Now that your gut is stronger and your microbiome is more in balance, you can add the following healthy foods back into your diet. The meal plans and recipes in Phase 2 reflect these choices.

Dairy

- Goat's or sheep's milk products of all types: milk, cheese, yogurt
- Kefir of all types, including cow's milk

However, if you react strongly to dairy, you can substitute coconut milk for kefir in the smoothie recipes, and you can simply leave out the cheese or yogurt.

Eggs

- Preferably organic, free-range, and Omega 3 fortified

Fruits

- Mango
- Melons of all types—except watermelon, which is too high in sugar content
- Peaches
- Pears

Gluten-Free Grains

- Amaranth

- Buckwheat (yes, wheat contains gluten, but buckwheat is gluten-free!)
- Millet
- Oats, if they have been produced in a facility that can keep them gluten-free, such as Bob's Red Mill
- Quinoa
- Rice: brown rice, basmati rice, wild rice. No white rice, which is too high in starch and has too few vital nutrients

Legumes

- Green beans
- Beans of all types: black, kidney, red, white

Vegetables

- Sweet potatoes, yams

PHASE 2: YOUR METABOLIC BOOST: FOUR WEEKS TO ACCELERATE YOUR METABOLISM

I have provided you with fourteen days' worth of meal plans. When you have finished those first two weeks, repeat them for the second two weeks. If you like, you can add any of the choices below to any of the meals or snacks:

- Salad with Lemon Vinaigrette (page 263), including any of the following ingredients: lettuce (except iceberg), watercress, asparagus, cucumber, red peppers, red or green onion. You can throw in one-quarter avocado if you like.
- Broccoli, broccolini, kale, collards, kohlrabi.
- Fermented foods: kimchee, sauerkraut, or fermented vegetables of your choice.
- The following snacks from the meal plan: Roasted Curried Cauliflower*, Kale Chips*, Sliced Jerusalem artichoke, Roasted Asparagus Spears*.

*DENOTES RECIPES PROVIDED

I'd like you to basically avoid alcohol in Phases 1 and 2 because of its potentially stressful impact on the microbiome. In Phase 3 you can include some alcoholic beverages as part of your 30 percent indulgence. In all three phases I advise limiting your caffeinated coffee intake to one or two eight-ounce cups per day and your caffeinated tea intake to three to five eight-ounce cups per day. You can have as much decaf coffee and herbal tea as you like. Please avoid fruit juices, which are the least healthy way to consume fruit—you really want the fiber along with the fructose! Vegetable juices can be healthy if they are fresh and really contain only veggies, but watch out for the commercially bottled ones, which usually have a high quantity of fruit juice. They may be "natural," as their labels proclaim, but they are not necessarily healthy, especially if you are trying to lose weight.

Your Microbiome Supersupplements

Take these supplements any time of day you like, with or without meals, unless otherwise specified.

To remove unhealthy bacteria from your intestines, you have two choices:

1. You can look for a combination product that contains the following ingredients:
   - Berberine
   - Wormwood
   - Caprylic acid
   - Grapefruit seed extract
   - Garlic
   - Oregano Oil

I have recommended a few good combination products in the Resources section. Just follow the directions on the bottle for dosage.

2. You can take a single product. Choose either:

- Garlic, 5000 micrograms, three times a day

OR

- Berberine, 200 mg, three times a day

To Replace Stomach Acid

- Hydrochloric acid, 1000 mg with each meal

OR

- Apple cider vinegar, 1 teaspoon diluted with 5 to 6 teaspoons of water, with each meal. Gradually increase the dose until you are drinking 3 to 4 teaspoons of vinegar with each meal.

To Replace Enzymes

Find a good combination production that includes:

- Protease, which digests protein
- Lipase, which digests fat
- Amylase, which digests starches
- DPP 41V, which helps digest gluten and casein (milk protein), in case trace elements end up in your meal

Take 1 to 2 pills per meal.

I have recommended some good combination products in Resources.

Reinoculate with Probiotics

1. Find a good probiotic with the following qualities:

- The more diverse species, the better
- Should contain at least these three types of *Lactobacillus*: *acidophilous, rameneses, planataris*
- Should contain different types of *Bifidobacter*
- A bonus is if it contains *Acidophilus reuterii*
- Should contain between 50 billion and 200 billion bacteria—the more, the better

Take one pill or packet a day. I have recommended some good brands in Resources.

2. For weight loss take *Acidophilus gasseri*, which you will have to buy separately unless you have purchased one of the few probiotics that contains it. I have recommended some sources in Resources. Take as directed.

Reinoculate with Prebiotics
1. Take inulin powder: 4 to 6 grams a day, divided into two doses
2. Take arabinogalactans, 500 to 1000 mg, two times a day

You can also look for a combination of inulin and arabinogala-catans. I have recommended some good combination products in Resources.

3. Take cal-mag butyrate, 200 to 300 mg, one to two times a day. Butyrate is both a prebiotic and a weight loss supplement.

When you look for supplements to repair the gut you'd do best to find a combination product, either in pill or powder form—I prefer powder. Some of the individual ingredients to look for include the following (or you can take them individually in the doses listed):

1. Glutamine: 1 to 5 grams a day
2. Quercitin: 100 to 500 mg a day; look for "iso-quercitin," which is better absorbed
3. Zinc alone or with carnosine. If in combination, 100 to 150 mg a day. If you take zinc by itself, take 30 mg a day, and then take carnosine in a dose of 100 to 500 mg a day.
4. N-acetyl glucosamine, 1000 mg a day
5. DGL (diglycerinated licorice), 400 mg a day

6. Slippery elm, 200 mg a day
7. Marshmallow 100 mg a day

You can also take a combination product. I recommend several in Resources.

Additional Weight Loss Aids

1. Meratrim: 400 mg, two times a day, thirty minutes before breakfast and dinner.
2. *Sphaeranthus indicus* and *Garcinia mangostana*. You can buy them separately and follow the directions on the bottle, or look for a formula that includes those compounds and meratrim. Some combinations include capsicum, which offers additional weight loss benefits, as well as zychrome, which helps to balance blood sugar. See Resources for some suggestions.
3. Green coffee bean extract, 400 mg, two times a day.
   OR
   Irvingia (African mango), 150 to 300 mg, two times a day

MEAL PLANS FOR THE METABOLIC BOOST

PHASE TWO

* DENOTES RECIPES PROVIDED

WEEK 1

DAY 1

BREAKFAST
Minted Fruit Salad with Brazil Nuts*

SNACK
Jicama and radish slices with almond butter

LUNCH
Gazpacho Smoothie*

SNACK
Spiced Roasted Chickpeas* (use leftover Spiced Roasted Chickpeas from Day 21 of Phase 1)

DINNER
Italian-Accented Chicken Stew,* Steamed Quinoa,* and green beans, 6 tablespoons your choice of fermented vegetables

DAY 2

BREAKFAST
Granola with Oats and Flaxseed Crumbles* with apple and coconut milk

SNACK
Tomato, cucumber, jicama, and endive leaves with Romesco*

LUNCH
Chèvre, Beets, and Jicama Salad*

SNACK
Roasted Asparagus with Lemon* (use leftover Roasted Asparagus from Phase 1, Day 19)

DINNER
Grilled Beef Burger with Grilled Portobello Mushroom Napoleon,* lettuce and tomato, 6 tablespoons your choice of fermented vegetable

MEAL PLANS FOR THE METABOLIC BOOST

DAY 3

BREAKFAST
Poached eggs on Avocado and Tomato topped with yogurt and chili oil or hot sauce*

SNACK
Apple slices with almond butter

LUNCH
Mango Smoothie*

SNACK
Roasted Sweet Potato Chips*

DINNER
Borscht* with green salad, 6 tablespoons your choice of fermented vegetables

DAY 4

BREAKFAST
Granola with Oats and Flaxseed Crumbles* with berries and coconut milk

SNACK
Vegetable medley—your choice—with pine nuts and Basil Pesto* (use the extra Basil Pesto* you made on Phase 1, Day 6)

LUNCH
Leek, Onion, and Potato Soup*

SNACK
Roasted Asparagus Spears with Lemon*

DINNER
Mexican Rice and Beans with Avocado and Mango*, mixed greens salad, 6 tablespoons your choice of fermented vegetables

MEAL PLANS FOR THE METABOLIC BOOST

DAY 5

BREAKFAST
Two hard-boiled eggs with tomato, radish, and asparagus

SNACK
Mango and apple slices with almond butter

LUNCH
Kale Salad à la Greque*

SNACK
"Baked" Apple Cider Smoothie*

DINNER
Italian-Accented Chicken Stew* (Use leftover Italian-Accented Chicken Stew from Phase 2, Day 1) over Steamed Quinoa* and green beans, 6 tablespoons your choice of fermented vegetables

DAY 6

BREAKFAST
Quinoa with Chopped Apples and Almonds*

SNACK
Half grapefruit with a dusting of cinnamon

LUNCH
Black Bean and Rice Salad* (use leftover Mexican Rice and Beans from Phase 2, Day 4), served with tomato on greens with Orange Cumin Vinaigrette*

SNACK
Curried Roasted Cauliflower*

DINNER
Brazilian Fish Stew*; 6 tablespoons your choice of fermented vegetables

MEAL PLANS FOR THE METABOLIC BOOST

WEEK 2

DAY 7

BREAKFAST
Scrambled Eggs with Leeks, Onions, and Tarragon*

SNACK
Mango Smoothie*

LUNCH
Apple Harvest Spinach Salad*

SNACK
Spiced Roasted Chickpeas* (use the leftover Spiced Roasted Chickpeas from Phase 2, Day 1)

DINNER
Greek-Inspired Beef Stew with Onion, Feta Cheese, and Walnuts*, 6 tablespoons your choice of fermented vegetables

DAY 8

BREAKFAST
Blueberry Kale Smoothie*

SNACK
Spiced Roasted Chickpeas* (Use leftover Spiced Roasted Chickpeas from Phase 2, Day 1)

LUNCH
Classic Greek Salad with Sheep's Milk Feta*

SNACK
Vegetable medley with Basil Pesto*

DINNER
Lamb Stew Provencal*, 6 tablespoons your choice of fermented vegetables

MEAL PLANS FOR THE METABOLIC BOOST

DAY 9

BREAKFAST

Frittata* with Swiss chard, onion, and potato

SNACK

Mango Smoothie*

LUNCH

Chèvre, Beets, and Jicama Salad*

SNACK

Parsnip, zucchini, and jicama sticks with Basil Pesto* (use the extra Basil Pesto* you made on Phase 1, Day 6)

DINNER

Fish Stew with Romesco*, Easy Sautéed Greens*, Steamed Quinoa*, 6 tablespoons your choice of fermented vegetables

DAY 10

BREAKFAST

Citrusy Avocado Compote*

SNACK

Escarole Chickpea Soup* (use the frozen Chicken Stock you made at the beginning of the diet)

LUNCH

Frittata* (Use the leftover Frittata from Phase 2, Day 9) and salad

SNACK

Baked apple with cinnamon (see the instructions in the Apple Harvest Spinach Salad* on page 260.)

DINNER

Chili Con Carne* with brown rice with mixed green salad, 6 tablespoons your choice of fermented vegetables

MEAL PLANS FOR THE METABOLIC BOOST

DAY 11

BREAKFAST
Granola with Oats and Flaxseed Crumbles* with fruit and coconut milk

SNACK
Jicama and radish slices with almond butter

LUNCH
Turkish-Style Cucumber Soup*

SNACK
Roasted Asparagus with Lemon*

DINNER
Borscht* (use leftover frozen Borscht from Phase 2, Day 3), with green salad, 6 tablespoons your choice of fermented vegetables

DAY 12

BREAKFAST
Hard-boiled eggs with tomato, cucumber, olives, and radish slices

SNACK
Guacamole Smoothie*

LUNCH
Green salad topped with leftover Fish Stew with Romesco*, Roasted Asparagus*, jicama, and tomato (use leftover Fish Stew with Romesco from Phase 2, Day 9 and the leftover Roasted Asparagus from Phase 2, Day 11)

SNACK
Sauerkraut and Meatball Soup (use the frozen soup you made from Phase 1, Day 4)

DINNER
Chili Con Carne* with brown rice (Use leftover Chili Con Carne from Phase 2, Day 10), 6 tablespoons your choice of fermented vegetables

MEAL PLANS FOR THE METABOLIC BOOST

DAY 13

BREAKFAST
"Baked" Apple Cider Smoothie*

SNACK
Curried Roasted Cauliflower*

LUNCH
Savory Pear Salad*

SNACK
Turkish-Style Cucumber Soup* (use leftover refrigerated Cucumber Soup from Phase 2, Day 11)

DINNER
Mussels Steamed in Beer* with Easy Sautéed Greens*, 6 tablespoons your choice of fermented vegetables

DAY 14

BREAKFAST
Poached Eggs on Avocado and Tomato*

SNACK
Sliced pear with almond butter

LUNCH
Apple Harvest Spinach Salad*

SNACK
Curried Roasted Cauliflower* (use leftover Curried Roasted Cauliflower from Day 13)

DINNER
Jerk Cornish Game Hen* with Mango Salsa*, steamed broccoli with lemon quarter and cooked millet, 6 tablespoons your choice of fermented vegetables

fourteen

PHASE 3:
YOUR LIFETIME TUNE-UP
TO MAINTAIN HEALTHY
WEIGHT FOR LIFE

B RAVO! NOW YOU HAVE COMPLETED THE FIRST SEVEN WEEKS OF THE Microbiome Diet. Your leaky gut is either completely healed or close to it. Your microbiome is now robust and healthy. If you have not yet reached your ideal weight, you should continue to lose weight by following this way of eating. If you have reached your ideal weight, you should be able to maintain it using this approach.

STAYING HEALTHY FOR LIFE

Now you are eating in synch with your inner ecology. Your own hungers and cravings have become a reliable guide for what your body needs. You no longer feel obsessed with foods that are unhealthy—perhaps you don't even desire those foods!

At this point you should listen to your body, identify what you are truly hungry for, and eat what you like. Of course, you are free to follow the meal plans from either phase of the Microbiome Diet, but you can experiment with your own combinations and assortments of food as well. Just be sure to keep loading up on Microbiome Super-foods and Superspices.

I'd like you to continue to practice stress-free eating, because that will make an enormous difference to your metabolism and to your pleasure in food. I'd also like you to ask yourself, always, what you are truly hungry for. If you really want food, enjoy your meal or snack! If you seek companionship, comfort, meaning, or some other good thing that is *not* food, please find another way to satisfy that hunger other than at the refrigerator.

Your Microbiome Supersupplements

At this point you have almost certainly removed the unhealthy bacteria from your system. However, you should continue to replace enzymes and stomach acid as needed, reinoculate with probiotics and prebiotics, and keep your gut wall in good repair. When you have lost all the weight you want you can stop taking the weight loss supplements.

To Replace Stomach Acid

- Hydrochloric acid, 1000 mg with each meal

OR

- Apple cider vinegar, 1 teaspoon diluted with 5 to 6 tea-spoons of water, with each meal. Gradually increase the dose until you are drinking 3 to 4 teaspoons of vinegar with each meal.

To Replace Enzymes

Find a good combination production that includes:

- Protease, which digests protein
- Lipase, which digests fat
- Amylase, which digests starches
- DPP 41V, which helps digest gluten and casein (milk protein) in case trace elements end up in your meal

Take 1 to 2 pills per meal.

I have recommended some good combination products in Resources.

Reinoculate with Probiotics

1. Find a good probiotic with the following qualities:

    - The more diverse species, the better
    - Should contain at least these three types of *Lactobacillus*: *acidophilous, rameneses, planataris*
    - Should contain different types of *Bifidobacter*
    - A bonus is if it contains *Acidophilus reuterii*
    - Should contain between 50 billion and 200 billion bacteria—the more, the better

    Take 1 pill or packet a day. I have recommended some good brands in Resources.

2. **Optional in Phase 3:** For weight loss take *Acidophilus gasseri*, which you will have to buy separately unless you have purchased one of the few probiotics that contains it. I have recommended some sources in Resources. Take as directed.

Reinoculate with Prebiotics

1. Take inulin powder, 4 to 6 grams a day, divided into two doses
2. Take arabinogalactans, 500 to 1000 mg, two times a day

You can also look for a combination of inulin and arabinogala-catans. I have recommended some good combination products in Resources.

3.　Take cal-mag butyrate, 200 to 300 mg, 1 to 2 times a day. Butyrate is both a prebiotic and a weight loss supplement.

When you look for supplements to repair the gut you'd do best to find a combination product, either in pill or powder form—I prefer powder. Some of the individual ingredients to look for include the following, or you can take them individually in the doses listed:

1.　Glutamine: 1 to 5 grams a day
2.　Quercitin: 100 to 500 mg a day; look for "iso-quercitin," which is better absorbed.
3.　Zinc alone or with carnosine. If in combination, 100 to 150 mg a day. If you take zinc by itself, take 30 mg a day, and then take carnosine in a dose of 100 to 500 mg a day.
4.　N-acetyl glucosamine, 1000 mg a day
5.　DGL (diglycerinated licorice), 400 mg a day
6.　Slippery elm, 200 mg a day
7.　Marshmallow 100 mg a day

You can also take a combination product. I recommend several in Resources.

Additional Weight Loss Aids: Optional in Phase 3

1.　Meratrim: 400 mg, 2 times a day, 30 minutes before breakfast and dinner
2.　*Sphaeranthus indicus* and *Garcinia mangostana*. You can buy them separately and follow the directions on the bottle, or look for a formula that includes those compounds and meratrim. Some combinations include capsicum, which offers additional weight loss benefits, as well as zychrome,

which helps to balance blood sugar. See Resources for some suggestions.

3. Green coffee bean extract, 400 mg, 2 times a day
    OR
    Irvingia (African mango), 150 to 300 mg, two times a day

70 PERCENT COMPLIANCE

You will continue to support both your gut and your microbiome with healing foods, probiotics, and prebiotics, but you should now be able to maintain only 70 percent compliance. The other 30 percent of the time you are free to eat almost anything you want. That means of the thirty-five meals and snacks you consume each week, about ten can include a food not on my "acceptable" list.

However, there are some foods that are so unhealthy that I would prefer you to avoid them as much as possible—all the time, if you are willing to do so! The following foods compromise your microbiome or your gut to a significant extent, so eat them at most two or three times a year—if that.

- Processed or packaged foods
- High-fructose corn syrup
- Trans fats
- Hydrogenated fats
- Canned fruits
- Fruit Juices
- Soy, including soy milk, soy sauce, tofu, tempeh, and all forms of soy isolate protein such as are found in many protein bars, protein shakes, and protein powders (check the label!), except soy lecithin
- Canola oil or cottonseed oil

Because of the way gluten can adversely affect your gut walls, I would also advise you to consume foods that contain gluten—bread, pasta, baked goods—no more than twice a week. Likewise, because of their grave risks to your health, I would advise you to consume sweeteners other than Lakanto no more than once or twice a week.

DISCOVERING YOUR POWER TO HEAL

As you can see, I have deliberately chosen not to create a maintenance plan that gives figures and formulas for how much you need and when you need it—no percentage of fats versus carbs, no portion sizes, no counting and measuring. That is because once you reset your metabolism and restore your gut health you won't need those kinds of guidelines. Every one of us is different, and we each need different things at different times. You have the ability to make healthy choices as guided by your microbiome and your "gut reactions." Now that you have experienced seven weeks on the Microbiome Diet you are in a position to know what feels good, what your body needs, and what choices are right for you, moment by moment, day by day, for the rest of your life.

Yes, you are the leader of your own inner ecology and responsible for its care. Armed with the knowledge you have gotten from this book and from your own experience of the past seven weeks, you will make wise decisions to maintain the health you've worked hard to achieve.

fifteen

YOUR PANTRY LIST, SHOPPING LISTS, AND TIME-SAVING STRATEGIES

PANTRY LIST FOR MICROBIOME DIET, PHASES 1 AND 2

Here are pantry staples and equipment you will use throughout Phases 1 and 2. Have these items on hand when you begin the Microbiome Diet. You can buy them ahead of time or when you pick up your first week's groceries. Some of these items can be bought online—see Resources for details.

Equipment

  1 small bowl
  1 10-cup bowl
  1 small saucepan
  1 medium saucepan with lid

1 small ovenproof casserole with lid
1 6-inch cast-iron pan
1 8-inch skillet
1 16-cup stock pot
12 x 18-inch sheet pan
13 x 18-inch sheet pan
1 steamer basket to fit medium saucepan with lid
assorted containers for refrigerating or freezing
12 2-cup freezer containers for soup stock
1 flat metal spatula
1 heavy-duty blender
1 large metal strainer
1 set measuring spoons
1 set measuring cups
1 grapefruit-sectioning spoon or knive
mandolin with safety guard
waterproof black marker, for marking leftovers you are refrig-
    erating or freezing

Foods

Nuts and nut butters

Nut butters:
organic almond butter
organic sunflower seed butter
Nuts (all should be raw, not roasted):
almonds
Brazil nuts
macadamia nuts
pine nuts
walnuts

Oils

coconut oil
flaxseed oil
olive oil
sunflower oil

Spices
cinnamon
cumin
curry powder
turmeric

Other items
apple cider, organic, nonsweetened, 1 gallon

beef stock, cans or cartons, organic (optional), 24 cups (package size varies by brand, but 32-ounce boxes are recommended; buy if you are not making your own Beef Base*.)

butter or organic ghee, 1 pound

chicken stock, cans or cartons, organic (optional), 13 cups (package size varies by brand, but 32-ounce boxes are recommended; buy if you are not making your own Chicken Base*.)

chickpeas, canned, organic, 9 15-ounce cans

dijon mustard, 1 10-ounce jar

fermented vegetables, 6 16-ounce jars (make sure no whey has been used in the fermentation process)

pea protein powder 1 8-ounce package

kimchee, 1 16-ounce jar

Lakanto 1 8-ounce package

rice flour, 3 ounces

sauerkraut (made without whey), 2 cups

SHOPPING LISTS FOR PHASE 1
Week 1
Fruits
3 apples
½ pint blueberries
3 grapefruits
5 kiwi fruits
3 lemons
1 lime

2 mangoes

1 ripe nectarine or ripe pear

6 oranges

½ pint raspberries

1 pint strawberries

Meats, Fish, and Shellfish

5 pounds beef bones (for Beef Base*)

3 pounds beef stew meat

1 6-pound chicken (for Chicken Base*)

1 pound boneless chicken breasts or thighs

½ pound chopped meat

7 ounces dry U-15 sea scallops

Miscellaneous

1 gallon unsweetened apple cider

1 32-ounce carton organic beef broth

2 32-ounce cartons organic chicken stock

1 12-ounce gluten-free bottle of beer

1 17-ounce bottle hot sauce (Frank's) or sriracha

8 ounces kalamata olives

3 ounces raw pine nuts

1 5-ounce can organic tomato paste

Vegetables and Herbs

½ pound asparagus

3 avocados

1 bunch basil leaves

6 carrots

1 head cauliflower

1 pint cherry tomatoes

1 bunch celery

3 cucumbers

1 bunch fresh dill

1 fennel

1 large head of garlic

1 ginger root (½ pound)

12 cups mixed greens
1 jicama
1 medium bunch kale
1 bunch fresh mint
½ pound button mushrooms
1 3-pound bag yellow onions
1 red onion
1 bunch parsley
4 parsnips
1 bunch radish
1 small red pepper
2 ounces snow peas
1 small bunch Swiss chard or escarole
1 small butternut squash
1 small spaghetti squash
4 ripe tomatoes
1 bunch watercress

Week 2

Fruits

6 large apples
½ pint blueberries
2 grapefruits
2 kiwis
2 lemons
1 lime
1 mango
3 ripe nectarines or pears
2 oranges

Meats, Fish, and Shellfish

1½ pounds chopped beef
1 pound chicken, boneless skinless breast or thighs
7 to 8 ounces cod
1 pound grouper, catfish or cod

1 pound lamb stew

1 pound mussels

Miscellaneous

1 12-ounce bottle gluten-free beer

1-pound bag dry lentils

1 32-ounce container coconut milk (unsweetened)

1 1-pound bag frozen green peas

3 ounces raw pine nuts

1 bag or can of organic sauerkraut (2 cups)

1 28-ounce can organic fire-roasted chopped tomatoes

1 750-ml bottle dry white wine

Vegetables and Herbs

2 artichokes

24 asparagus

2 avocados

1 bunch arugula

1 bunch fresh basil

1 head broccoli rabe or escarole

1 small green head cabbage

3 carrots

1 bunch cilantro

1 head cauliflower

1 medium eggplant

1 small fennel bulb

8 cups greens

2 bunches kale

1 leek

1 bunch fresh mint

¾ pound mushrooms

7 large button or cremini or small Portobello mushrooms

2 medium Portobello mushrooms

1 parsnip

1 green pepper

1 jalapeno pepper

1 sweet red pepper

1 small butternut squash
1 small spaghetti squash
1 large bunch spinach
1 large turnip
2 small turnips

Week 3

Fruits

1 apple
1 pint blueberries
2 grapefruits
3 kiwis
2 lemons
2 mangos
1 nectarine
2 oranges
½ pint strawberries

Vegetables and Herbs

1 artichoke
18 asparagus
1 avocado
1 small bunch carrots
1 bunch celery
1 cucumber
2 fennel bulbs
6 cups greens, your choice of the following: mesclun greens, which might also be labeled field greens or assorted baby greens; red oak leaf lettuce; red leaf lettuce; arugula; baby spinach; Romaine lettuce; bibb lettuce; Belgian endive; or any lettuces of your choice (except iceberg)
1-pound bag Jerusalem artichokes
1 jicama
1 bunch kale
6 button mushrooms
1 red pepper

6 radishes
4 stalks Swiss chard
1 tomato
½ pint cherry tomatoes
1 cup watercress

SHOPPING LISTS FOR PHASE 2
Week 1

Fruits

3 apples
1 pint berries, your choice
2 grapefruits
2 kiwis
5 mangos
2 oranges

Meat, Fish, and Shellfish

½ pound ground beef
3 pounds beef stew
1 pound skinless and boneless chicken breast or thighs
7 ounces cod

Miscellaneous

1 15-ounce can organic black beans
1 15-ounce can organic white beans
6 ounces fresh creamy-style chèvre (goat's milk cheese)
2 12-ounce cans organic chickpeas (garbanzos)
32 ounces coconut milk (unsweetened)
6 eggs
8 ounces sheep's or goat's milk feta cheese
16 ounces flaxseed
32 ounces gluten-free oats (Bob's Red Mill)
1 quart goat's or sheep's milk kefir
24 ounces quinoa
1 cup organic brown rice
1 cup sunflower seeds

2 cups goat's or sheep's milk yogurt

1 750-ml bottle red wine

Vegetables and Herbs

12 asparagus

3 avocados

2 small beets and 8 large beets

2 heads cauliflower

1 small celeriac (celery root)

2 cucumbers

1 endive

1 small romaine lettuce

1 small bibb lettuce

1 small head escarole

1 large head of garlic

6 green beans

6 cups salad greens

2 jicama

1 big bunch kale

2 leeks

2 Portobello mushrooms, 4 inches in diameter

7 large white or cremini mushrooms, 2 inches in diameter

1 red onion

3 yellow onions

1 jalapeño pepper

3 white potatoes

4 radishes

1 small bunch spinach

4 ripe tomatoes or 4 cherry tomatoes and 4 regular tomatoes

2 tomatillos

2 large sweet potatoes

1 bunch cilantro

Week 2

Fruits

4 apples

2 grapefruits
1 kiwi
1 lime
3 mangos
2 oranges
2 pears

Meats, Fish, and Shellfish
1 pound chopped beef
1 Cornish game hen
7 ounces grouper, cod, or catfish
½ pound lamb stew
1 pound Prince Edward Island mussels (about 15)

Miscellaneous
1 12-ounce bottle of gluten-free beer
¼ pound sheep's or goat's milk blue cheese
½ pound sheep's milk feta cheese
¼ pound pecorino Romano cheese
2 15-ounce cans organic chickpeas
1 15-ounce can organic red kidney beans
1 15-ounce can organic white beans
1 quart goat's or sheep's milk kefir
2 cups sheep's or goat milk yogurt
½ cup brown rice

Vegetables and Herbs
12 asparagus
1 avocado
1 beet
1 small head broccoli
2 carrots
3 cucumbers
2 bunches dill
21 bunches escarole
10 cups mixed green salad
12 green beans

1 small bunch kale

2 bunches mint

3 large mushrooms for stuffing

1 parsnip

2 potatoes

2 ounces snow peas

1 small bunch of spinach

1 small bunch Swiss chard

2 tomatoes

1 small zucchini

WEEKLY WORK PLANS

Use these work plans to organize your work as you prepare food ahead of time on Sundays and as you put leftovers aside for use during the week. If you can't or don't want to follow these exact plans, try to choose one day a week (a weekend day or evening is great) to make some of the dishes that are more time-consuming. Of course, you can also do some of the preparations in the evening or while some of the frozen dinners are being heated. Making double batches and freezing in smaller portions is a great way to make sure you always have microbiome-supporting meals at the ready, even when you don't have time to cook. For your convenience these time-savers are built right into the meal plans.

One huge time-saver concerns the Beef Base* (page 278) and Chicken Base* (page 289): you can make everything you need for both phases on your first day of cooking and freeze it to reheat later. That means you'll be making homemade soups in about half an hour. If you prefer, you can buy organic beef or chicken stock (it's on your shopping list as an option), but I think you'll enjoy the home-made more, and you'll definitely get more nourishment from it.

Carefully seal all prepared foods and mark each container with the name of the recipe and the date. Keep a list of all the frozen and refrigerated foods and mark them off when used.

PHASE 1

WEEK 1

Sunday preceding Day 1

1. Prepare the chicken soup base recipe. Reserve enough for Day 2 lunch and the lemon chicken recipe, and divide the remainder into 1- or 2-cup containers, and freeze for future use.
2. Prepare the lemon chicken.
3. Prepare beef stock for sauerkraut soup. Prepare meatballs for the soup. Freeze half of the meatballs for the Meatballs with Roasted Spaghetti Squash and Basil Pesto entrée. Freeze the stock in 2-cup freezer containers.
4. Roast the spaghetti squash; seed and shred the flesh. Refrigerate.
5. Make the basil pesto.

WEEK 2

Sunday

1. Make the Curried Lamb and Lentil Stew.
2. Make the Rich Vegetable Soup.
3. Make the Beef Stew with Aromatic Vegetables and Red Wine.
4. Make the Braised Apple Chicken.
5. Char cook the eggplant for Rumanian Eggplant Salad.

WEEK 3

Sunday

1. Make chicken bone broth, and freeze in 2-cup containers.
2. Make Borscht, and freeze in 2-cup containers.

PHASE 2

WEEK 1

Sunday and/or Weekday Evening

1. Make Granola with Oats and Flaxseed Crumbles.
2. Make Italian-Accented Chicken Stew.
3. Cook Mexican Beans and Rice. Refrigerate separately. Make Mango Salsa.
4. Make Leek, Onion, and Potato Soup.

WEEK 2

Sunday and/or Weekday Evening

1. Make Greek-Inspired Beef Stew.
2. Make Lamb Stew Provencal.
3. Make Chili Con Carne.
4. Make Steamed Quinoa
5. Make jerk rub (see Jerk Cornish Game Hen).

WEEK 3

Sunday

1. Make chicken bone broth, and freeze in 2-cup containers.
2. Make Borscht, and freeze in 2-cup containers.

sixteen

RECIPES

I AM EXCITED TO SHARE WITH YOU THE WONDERFUL MEAL PLANS AND recipes created by wellness chef Carole Clark. Chef Carole worked closely with me to embody the principles of the Microbiome Diet in delicious recipes that will feed your senses, heal your gut, and rebalance your microbiome.

Each recipe notes which phase it is suited for. Most of these recipes can be prepared in half an hour or less. A few require some advance prep time, but either that can be done on Sundays or weekday evenings when you are doing your advance preparation. Carole has created a work plan for each phase of the diet (see Work Plans on page 243) based on you investing a few hours each Sunday to prepare food for the week ahead. It might take somewhat longer the first couple of times you try it, but as you get used to it, you'll be able to complete the "advance prep" more quickly. That way you have at most half an hour—and sometimes far less—to prepare or heat up each meal during the week. As noted, you can make all of the Beef Base* (page 278) and Chicken Base* (page 289) for the entire diet the first time you prepare food—just freeze in two-cup containers and then reheat.

I know the latest trend for busy cooks is sautéing, roasting, and other quick methods of preparing food. However, I deeply believe that for healing the gut, soups and stews are far superior. You get more nutrients, the warm liquids are soothing and easily absorbed, and you are generally choosing a healthier means of cooking. So please, invest a few hours each Sunday in your gut health, your microbiome, and your ability to lose weight. Your reward will be delicious, satisfying food; freedom from cravings and outsized appetite; and healthy, permanent weight loss. Plus, in three weeks you can enjoy extra indulgences 10 percent of the time, and at the end of seven weeks you can eat indulgently 30 percent of the time. I hope a few hours of meal prep on Sunday night seems like a fair exchange!

I chose to work with a chef of Carole's caliber because I want you to enjoy every bite you put into your mouth! As you will see in Chapters 7 and 8, savoring the tastes, textures, and aromas of the food you eat will help you switch from the "fight or flight" portion of your nervous system to that part of your anatomy that is dedicated to "rest and digest." Stress-free eating is an important aspect of the Microbiome Diet, and what better way to destress than to sit down to a delicious meal full of rich, satisfying flavors? These recipes are easy to prepare, but because of Carole's creative use of ingredients, you will get maximum pleasure from every meal.

PHASE 1

BREAKFASTS

"BAKED" APPLE CIDER SMOOTHIE

You can either bake the apple or use a raw one. Either way, the spices make the whole thing taste like your favorite apple dessert. Even though this is a superhealthy way to start your morning—with protein, probiotic kefir, and a vitamin-rich apple—this breakfast smoothie will make you feel as though you're having dessert.

1 SERVING

1 small raw apple, peeled, seeded, cored, and chunked, about 1 cup, or 1 large baked apple, peeled, seeded, and cored (See directions for baking an apple in the Apple Harvest Spinach Salad,* page 260.)

¼ cup unsweetened apple cider

¼ cup kefir

1 small pear, peeled, seeded, cored, and chunked, about ¾ cup

2 tablespoons protein powder

½ teaspoon cinnamon

⅛ teaspoon nutmeg

⅛ teaspoon clove

3 ice cubes

1. Put all ingredients in a blender and liquefy.

BERRY, NECTARINE, KIWI, AND ORANGE MINTED FRUIT SALAD WITH CINNAMON

PHASE 1

This sweet-and-tart fruit salad is a delicious and refreshing way to start the day. For an extra healthy bonus, enjoy the fiber in the kiwi as well as cinnamon, which helps to balance your blood sugar and prevent insulin resistance.

1 SERVING

½ orange, cut in half through center, not stem end

1 ripe nectarine

¼ cup berries

1 big pinch of ground cinnamon

1 tablespoon fresh mint

1. Section orange, squeeze the shells, and reserve the juice.

2. Peel the nectarine and cut it into ½-inch slices. It should be juicy, so save the juice and add it to the orange juice. Add the nectarine slices to the orange sections.

3. Add the berries to the fruit mixture.

4. Add the cinnamon to the mixed juices, pour on top of the fruit, sprinkle with the mint, and serve.

PHASE 2

BLUEBERRY KALE SMOOTHIE

Invigorating! The robust flavor of the frozen blueberries masks the taste of the kale, even as this "silent" ingredient delivers valuable vitamins and nutrients. The avocado and almond butter feed your brain and your cells with healthy fats, the kefir is a natural probiotic, and the protein powder fuels your energy for a vigorous start to your day. A great way to get more greens into your diet while enjoying the sweet, tangy taste of blueberries and cider or kefir.

1 SERVING

½ cup chopped kale, ribs removed

½ cup frozen unsweetened organic blueberries

¼ avocado

1 teaspoon almond butter

¾ cup apple cider or kefir

5 ice cubes

2 tablespoons pea protein powder

1. Place all ingredients in a blender and process until smooth.

CITRUS BERRY SALAD WITH BRAZIL NUTS PHASE 1

This citrusy salad is a great way to get a huge dose of immune-protective vitamin C to start your morning. The kiwi is rich in microbiome-nourishing fiber, and the Brazil nuts add a serving of protein plus a nice portion of gut-healing Omega 3 fats. Quick, easy, delicious, and healthy—an energizing start to your day.

1 SERVING

½ grapefruit, cut in half through the center, not the stem end

1 orange

½ kiwi fruit

¼ cup blueberries or raspberries

⅛ cup fresh mint leaves

6 Brazil nuts

1. Section the grapefruit with a sectioning spoon or with a knife or regular spoon if you don't have a sectioning spoon. Squeeze the grapefruit shell for residual juice, and save it in a cup.

2. Cut the orange in half through the center, not the stem end, and section it. Squeeze the shells, and add the juice to the grapefruit juice. Add orange sections to the grapefruit sections.

3. Cut the kiwi in half, peel it, and slice it into ¼-inch slices. Add to the grapefruit and orange sections.

4. Add the berries to the fruit, and mix.

5. Add chopped mint leaves to the juices, and pour juice mixture over the fruit.

6. Serve the nuts on the side.

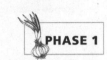

CITRUSY AVOCADO COMPOTE

Grapefruit and avocado is one of my favorite combinations—if you've never tried it, you're in for a treat! In this case the sharp, citrusy tastes of the orange and the sweetness of the kiwi are an added bonus. Plus you get loads of antioxidants, vitamin C, microbiome-nourishing fiber, and healthy fats for a delicious, healthy way to start the day.

1 SERVING

1 orange, halved through the center, not the stem end

½ grapefruit, cut in half through center, not stem end

½ kiwi

½ avocado (see below for slicing instructions)

1. Section the grapefruit with a sectioning spoon, or, if you don't have one, with a knife or regular spoon. Squeeze the grapefruit shell for residual juice, and save the juice in a cup.

2. Section the orange, squeeze the shells, and add the juice to the grapefruit juice. Add the orange sections to the grapefruit sections.

3. Cut the kiwi in half through the center, peel it, and slice it into ¼-inch slices. Add to the grapefruit and orange sections.

4. Peel the avocado, and remove half from the pit. Keep the pit attached to the half you are reserving for later use, wrapping it airtight. Slice the avocado, and add it to the fruit sections.

5. Pour the juices over the fruit mixture, and serve.

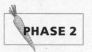

FRITTATA

You can definitely enjoy this frittata in the morning, but it also works beautifully for lunch or dinner, especially when served with a salad. You'll find suggested vegetables in this recipe, but feel free to improvise—what are *your* favorites? In this version the onions are a Microbiome Superfood that will nourish your microbiome while healing your gut, and the leafy greens offer you iron and B vitamins for stamina and stress reduction.

2 SERVINGS

6 organic eggs

2 tablespoons cold water

1 teaspoon snipped tarragon

¼ cup grated "goat" Parmesan, or Pecorino Romano, a sheep's milk cheese, divided

½ teaspoon salt

½ teaspoon pepper

1 cup sliced onions

2 tablespoons olive oil

1 small zucchini, cut into 1-inch slices

½ pound spinach or Swiss chard

Salt and pepper to taste

1. Preheat oven to 475°F.

2. Beat the eggs in a small bowl with cold water. Add tarragon, 2 tablespoons cheese, ½ teaspoon each salt and pepper, and combine. Set aside.

3. Sauté the onions over medium heat in an ovenproof nonstick 6-inch skillet in oil until translucent, about 5 minutes. Add zucchini, and sauté until lightly browned, about 7 minutes. Then add spinach, and cook until wilted, about 7 minutes.

4. Spread the vegetables evenly in the skillet. Season with salt and pepper. The pan should be hot. Pour the egg mixture over the vegetables, and cook until the eggs begin to set.

5. Sprinkle on 2 tablespoons cheese. Place the skillet in the hot oven, and bake for 5 minutes until the frittata is firm but not brown.

GRANOLA WITH OATS AND FLAXSEED CRUMBLES

PHASE 2

This is a filling, fast, and easy breakfast you can also munch on for a snack. To add a sweet note, eat it like cereal with coconut milk, and to make it even sweeter substitute unsweetened apple cider for the water. The flaxseed, almonds, almond butter, and coconut oil give you lots of healthy fats for cell and brain health, while the cinnamon helps to balance your blood sugar. This recipe makes enough for a few weeks and will keep so long as you store it in an airtight container in the fridge to preserve the flaxseed.

7 HALF-CUP SERVINGS

FOR THE FLAXSEED CRUMBLES

½ teaspoon cinnamon

¼ teaspoon allspice

½ teaspoon vanilla extract

1 cup water

1½ cups flaxseed

1 cup raw sunflower seeds

1. Combine the spices, vanilla, and water. Add the flaxseed, and let it rest for about 6 hours or, if you prefer, overnight. It should have an oily texture.

2. Spread the mixture evenly on a 12 x 18-inch sheet pan.

3. Bake in a preheated 275°F oven for 1 hour, stirring frequently. Remove from the oven, and let cool. When the mixture is still warm, break up any clumps. When cool, mix in sunflower seeds. Reserve.

FOR THE OATS

½ teaspoon allspice

½ teaspoon freshly ground nutmeg

1 teaspoon cinnamon

1 tablespoon vanilla extract

½ cup water

¼ cup coconut oil

2 tablespoons almond butter

1 cup sliced raw almonds

2 cups gluten-free rolled oats

1. Preheat oven to 300°F.

2. In a saucepan, add the spices and vanilla to the combined water, coconut oil, and almond butter, and cook on low for 2 minutes. Let cool.

3. In a medium bowl, mix the cooled liquid into the oats and nuts.

4. Put the mixture in a 12 x 18-inch sheet pan. Bake at 300°F for 30 minutes, stirring frequently. The mixture should be crispy.

5. Remove from the oven, and let cool.

6. Mix with the flaxseed mixture.

HARD-BOILED EGGS WITH TOMATO, RADISH, AND ASPARAGUS

PHASE 2

This is a lively way to dress up good old-fashioned hard-boiled eggs, not to mention using three Microbiome Superfoods to nourish your microbiome and help heal your gut. By the way, older eggs peel better than fresh ones, and to make a quicker breakfast you can even boil the eggs the day before you make the dish.

1 SERVING

2 organic eggs

4 asparagus, stem end removed

3 tomato slices

3 radishes, sliced in half

1. Place eggs in a heavy-bottomed saucepan and cover them with cold water. Cover the tops of the eggs with at least 1 inch of water. Bring the water to a full boil, uncovered. When there are very big bubbles, remove the pot from the heat

and cover it. Let the pot stand untouched for 15 minutes. Remove the boiled eggs from the water, and transfer them to a bowl of cold water for 10 minutes to stop the cooking process. Peel the egg, and slice into quarters.

2. Place water in a saucepan fitted with a steamer strainer. Fill with water to the bottom of the strainer. Heat to boiling, and turn down the heat to simmer. Place the asparagus in the steamer pan set. Steam for 5 to 10 minutes, depending on the thickness of the asparagus, or until asparagus is tender.

3. Assemble the eggs with the asparagus, tomato slices, and radishes on a plate, and serve.

MANGO SMOOTHIE   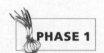 PHASE 1   PHASE 2

The tropical taste of mango and the zing of fresh ginger make a naturally sweet treat that will leave you feeling full, energized, and ready to start your day. Mango will boost your digestion as well as offer a fantastic source of vitamins A, C, and E along with folic acid and calcium. Ginger is good for your digestion and helps fight inflammation. And when you can add kefir in Phase 2, you are including a natural probiotic that will support your microbiome.

Because of the large flat seed inside, peeling and slicing a mango can be challenging, but because you're throwing it all in the blender, you don't have to worry about how it looks. Be prepared for a little mess— and an absolutely delicious taste.

If you've never cooked with fresh ginger before, you're in for a treat. It tastes about as different from powdered ginger as fresh peaches do from canned. Look for the small, brown, knobby root in the produce section. Peel off the thin skin and slice up the yellowish meat inside. Because you're throwing it all in the blender, don't worry about size or shape—just make them small enough to buzz.

1 SERVING

1 cup very ripe mango, peeled, seeded, chunked

½ cup cider, or, in Phase 2, kefir

¼ cup water

1 cup apple, peeled, cored, chunked

½ teaspoon chopped fresh ginger (optional)

2 tablespoons pea protein powder

3 ice cubes

1. Process all ingredients in a blender until smooth.

Minted Fruit Salad with Brazil Nuts   PHASE 1

This refreshing fruit salad is loaded with antioxidants, nutrients that help protect your body from oxidative stress as well as supporting your immune system. Plus the contrast between the sweet mango, the citrusy orange, and the tart berries makes for such a satisfying combination. You also get gut-healing Omega 3 healthy fats from the Brazil nuts.

1 SERVING

½ orange, cut in half through center, not stem end

½ ripe mango, sliced (see below for instructions)

1 teaspoon lime juice

¼ cup berries

1 tablespoon chopped fresh mint

8 Brazil nuts

1. Cut the orange in half through the center, not the stem end, and section it. Squeeze the shells, and reserve the juice.

2. A mango has a large flat seed in the center. Assume it is about ¾ inch thick. Cut the mango lengthwise along the long axis on one side of this seed. Make light cross-cut slices on the cut half. Be careful not to slice through the skin. Wrap the uncut half airtight, and refrigerate.

3. With your fingers, push the skin side of the mango cheek up, and your cross-cut surface will fan out. With a small knife cut off these chunks. Scrape the remaining flesh and juice into the orange juice.

4. Combine the lime juice with the orange-mango juice mixture. Add the berries and chopped mint.

5. Place in a serving bowl, and serve the Brazil nuts on the side.

NECTARINE KIWI SMOOTHIE

PHASE 1

In the summer you can enjoy the sweet, slightly tart taste of fresh nectarine. Off season, substitute a ripe pear. The combination of either fruit with the kiwi will wake up your taste buds with a delicate, intriguing flavor. Both pears and kiwis are Microbiome Superfoods that are natural prebiotics, nourishing your microbiome and also helping your gut to heal.

1 SERVING

1 large ripe nectarine or pear

1 kiwi, peeled

½ cup apple cider

1 teaspoon almond butter

2 tablespoons pea protein powder

3 ice cubes

½ teaspoon Lakanto or more to taste

1. Put all ingredients in a blender, and liquefy until smooth.

POACHED EGGS ON AVOCADO AND TOMATO

PHASE 2

This elegant dish is actually quite quick and simple to make, and it's one of the healthiest ways I know to enjoy eggs. You get some healthy fats with the avocado, a Microbiome Superfood with the tomato, and some probiotics in the yogurt topping. Plus the combination of tangy yogurt, piquant hot sauce, acid tomato, and creamy avocado is just fabulous with poached eggs.

When you make this dish use only very fresh eggs. Check the date on the container to make sure they are less than a week old.

1 SERVING

⅓ cup sheep's or goat's milk yogurt

¼ teaspoon salt

3 thick slices ripe tomato, cut into ½-inch chunks

¼ avocado, peeled and sliced into ½-inch chunks

2 large, very fresh organic eggs, at room temperature

2 drops hot sauce or more to taste

Salt and pepper to taste

1. Mix the yogurt with the salt in a small serving bowl, and top with the tomato and avocado.

2. Crack each egg into a small cup or bowl. If a yolk breaks, discard it.

3. Fill a pan with water. Use a pan that is at least 3 inches deep so there is enough water to cover the eggs. Bring the water to a boil, and then lower the heat to a simmer. If the water is too cool, the egg will separate apart before it cooks; if the water is too hot, you will end up with tough whites and an over-cooked yolk.

4. Set a timer for exactly 3 minutes for medium-firm yolks. Adjust the time up or down for runnier or firmer yolks. Cook 2½ to 5 minutes, depending on firmness desired.

5. Remove the eggs from the hot water with a slotted spoon. Lift each poached egg from the water, holding it over the pan briefly to let any water clinging to the egg drain off. Place each well-drained egg on the the tomato mixture. Add the hot sauce and salt and pepper to taste.

QUINOA WITH CHOPPED APPLE AND ALMONDS

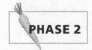

PHASE 2

We usually think of quinoa as savory, not sweet, but when you add the fruit and nuts, you've got a fabulous high-protein alternative to oatmeal. Almonds and flaxseed provide healthy fats for your cells and brain, while cinnamon helps balance your blood sugar. Grated ginger adds kick to the mix, plus some digestive health benefits and anti-inflammatory properties. This cereal will leave you feeling energized and satisfied but not stuffed or bloated.

1 SERVING

½ cup quinoa, rinsed and drained

1 cup water

⅛ teaspoon freshly grated nutmeg

½ cinnamon stick

1 teaspoon grated ginger root

1 tablespoon flaxseed oil

⅓ cup chopped apple

¼ cup coconut milk

Salt to taste

1 tablespoon chopped almonds

1. Stir the quinoa, water, nutmeg, cinnamon, ginger, and oil in a small pot. Heat to a boil. Reduce the heat, and simmer for 10 minutes.

2. Stir in the apple and coconut milk, and simmer for 5 minutes, until liquid is absorbed.

3. Salt to taste. Sprinkle on the nuts, and serve.

SCRAMBLED EGGS WITH LEEKS, ONIONS, AND TARRAGON

 PHASE 2

Who doesn't love the warm, comforting taste of scrambled eggs? And they're even better when they are enlivened with leeks, onions, and tarragon—a wonderful way to add flavor as well as two Microbiome Superfoods. You can make this dish quickly for a hot, filling breakfast that will help you power through your morning—so enjoy!

1 SERVING

2 fresh organic eggs

1 tablespoon cold water

1 teaspoon fresh, chopped tarragon, divided

1 tablespoon unsalted clarified butter or 1 tablespoon olive oil plus

1 tablespoon chopped leeks

2 tablespoons chopped onion

1 teaspoon clarified butter

Salt and pepper to taste

1. Break the eggs into a small bowl. Add the cold water, and whisk vigorously. Add ½ teaspoon tarragon.

2. Heat the tablespoon of unsalted clarified butter, and then sauté the leeks in it on medium-low heat for 2 minutes. Add the onion, and cook for 5 minutes until soft and golden.

3. Add the teaspoon of clarified butter, and place on medium heat until the butter bubbles. Pour the eggs into the middle of the pan. Stir slowly with a silicone spatula. As soon as curds (big soft lumps) begin to form, lower the heat to low, and fold the curds over on themselves. As soon as the egg is no longer liquid transfer the scramble onto the serving plate. Salt and pepper to taste.

SUNRISE SMOOTHIE

PHASE 1

This fruit combination makes a delicious sweet start to your day. Ginger is a terrific support for your digestion as well as a natural anti-inflammatory. The fruits are loaded with vitamins, and the almond butter gives you a serving of healthy fat to support cell and brain health. And it's loaded with protein powder to boost your energy.

For instructions on how to buy and prepare the ginger, see the recipe for Mango Smoothie, page 254. If fresh strawberries are not in season, buy frozen organic berries and just throw them into the blender without defrosting. If nectarines are out of season, an apple makes a good substitute.

1 SERVING

4 large ripe strawberries

1 large orange, squeezed

1 ripe nectarine or ½ apple, peeled and pitted

3 ice cubes

½ cup unsweetened apple cider

½ teaspoon peeled, finely chopped fresh ginger root
   (optional)

1 teaspoon almond butter

2 tablespoons pea protein powder

¼ teaspoon Lakanto (optional)

1. Put all ingredients in blender, and process until smooth.

LUNCHES

APPLE HARVEST SPINACH SALAD

PHASE 2

This salad is especially delicious in autumn during the apple harvest, when Jerusalem artichokes are the sweetest. Another root vegetable, celeriac, also called celery root, is part of the vegetable mix. Found in the produce section of the market, celeriac is a large, round, knobby root ball with hairy roots growing on it. It has a bright, piquant, clean taste, reminiscent of celery. Peel the thin skin and dice just before using.

When you make this salad you'll probably end up with some extra vinaigrette, which you can store in the fridge for future use.

This recipe is inspired by a lovely salad that's on the menu at Crossroads Food Shop, David Wurth's restaurant in Hillsdale, New York.

2 SERVINGS

1 apple, cored, with ½ inch of peel removed from the
   top of the apple

4 tablespoons water

1 small pinch cinnamon

1½ teaspoons Dijon mustard

⅓ cup apple cider vinegar

⅔ cup olive oil

¼ teaspoon salt

¼ teaspoon pepper

4 cups torn spinach leaves, washed and dried

½ cup sliced Jerusalem artichokes

½ cup peeled, diced celeriac

¼ cup goat's or sheep's milk feta cheese

Salt and pepper to taste

1. Preheat oven to 400°F.

2. Place the apple in a baking dish with the water. Put a pinch of cinnamon on the top of the apple. Bake for 25 to 30 minutes or until tender, not mushy. Let cool.

3. To make the vinaigrette, put the mustard and vinegar in a food processor, and pulse to blend. Add the oil in a slow, steady stream. Add the salt and pepper.

4. Peel, quarter, and cut the apple into small chunks. Place the spinach in a shallow bowl. Add the apple, Jerusalem artichokes, celeriac, and feta. Toss with 3 tablespoons of the vinaigrette. Add salt and pepper to taste.

PHASE 1

ARUGULA SALAD

This piquant salad wakes up your taste buds with its many contrasts in taste and texture: peppery arugula, sweet mango, smooth avocado, crunchy jicama, and zesty onion. The jicama and onion are Microbiome Superfoods. The avocado feeds your cells and supports your brain with healthy fats, while the arugula loads you up with stamina-building iron and stress-busting B vitamins. The mango is full of digestive enzymes that support the Replace step in the Four Rs (see Chapter 4).

2 SERVINGS

CITRUS VINAIGRETTE

1 tablespoon cider vinegar

Juice of ½ orange, about 3 tablespoons

Juice of 1 lime, about 2 tablespoons

½ teaspoon Dijon mustard

4 tablespoons olive oil

¼ teaspoon cumin

Salt and pepper

FOR THE SALAD

3 cups arugula leaves

½ avocado, peeled and sliced

½ mango, peeled and cut into slices (for instruction on
    how to cut the mango, see page 255)

¼ cup diced, peeled jicama

¼ red onion, thinly sliced

Salt and pepper to taste

Chicken slices (optional)

1. For the vinaigrette, whisk the vinegar and juices with the mustard. Slowly add
the oil. Add the cumin and salt and pepper.

2. Toss the arugula leaves with half of the vinaigrette.

3. Add the avocado, mango, jicama, and onion to the arugula mix, and salt and
pepper to taste. Add the chicken (optional).

4. Drizzle the remaining vinaigrette on top. Serve immediately. If you are taking
this salad to work, save this last step for just before you start to eat.

ASPARAGUS SALAD WITH LEMON VINAIGRETTE

PHASE 1

Asparagus, a Microbiome Superfood, has amazing anti-inflammatory
properties and is an excellent prebiotic. In this nutritious salad you get a
second Microbiome Superfood, the Jerusalem artichoke, or, if you can't
find that vegetable in your produce section, go for the jicama, also a
Microbiome Superfood. Both choices have a crisp texture and a sweet,
nutty taste. Get your share of healthy fats from the creamy avocado, a
delicious way to support cell health and brain function.

2 SERVINGS

FOR THE SALAD

½ pound asparagus, stems trimmed

½ cup water

2 tablespoons olive oil

¼ teaspoon salt

1 large Jerusalem artichoke or ¼ jicama, peeled and cut into ⅛-inch slices

½ ripe avocado, cut into ¼-inch slices

2 ounces snow peas, diagonally cut into ½-inch pieces

¼ pound mixed greens

2 teaspoons snipped fresh tarragon

LEMON VINAIGRETTE

2 tablespoons fresh lemon juice

1 teaspoon fined grated lemon zest

¼ teaspoon salt

½ teaspoon Dijon mustard

3 tablespoons olive oil

Kosher salt and pepper to taste

1. Place the asparagus in a large sauté pan, add the water, drizzle with oil, and season with salt. Simmer over medium heat. Reduce the heat to low, cover the pan with a lid, and simmer until the asparagus is just knife-tender, about 5 to 6 minutes. Remove the asparagus, and set aside until cool enough to handle.

2. For the vinaigrette, combine the lemon juice and zest in a small, nonreactive bowl (glass, stainless steel, or plastic). Season with salt. Add Dijon mustard and whisk. Slowly add the olive oil. Taste and season with additional salt and pepper or lemon juice as needed.

3. Cut the cooled asparagus into 1-inch pieces and place in a large bowl. Add Jerusalem artichoke, avocado, and snow peas; toss gently with the vinaigrette. Place the vegetables on the mixed greens, sprinkle with the snipped tarragon, and serve.

BEET, RICE, AND ORANGE SALAD
WITH ORANGE VINAIGRETTE

PHASE 2

These earthy beets, crunchy Jerusalem artichokes, and sweet oranges make a lively combination. The Jerusalem artichokes are a Microbiome Superfood, and the vinaigrette supplies you with lots of healthy fats for your brain and cell health.

You'll probably have some leftover vinaigrette after you're done, which is delicious with grilled fish and, of course, other salads.

1 SERVING

ORANGE VINAIGRETTE

1½ teaspoons Dijon mustard

¼ cup fresh orange juice

2 tablespoons apple cider vinegar

¼ cup olive oil

1 tablespoon flaxseed oil

1 teaspoon chopped orange zest

1 teaspoon chopped tarragon

Salt and pepper to taste

FOR THE SALAD

1 medium beet, roasted or boiled, cut into ½-inch dice

½ cup cooked wild or brown rice

2 Jerusalem artichokes, washed, dried, and diced

6 green beans, washed, trimmed, and cut into half-inch pieces

Salt and pepper to taste

1 large orange, washed, dried, peeled, deseeded, and cut into halved sections

2 cups mixed greens

1. To make the vinaigrette, whisk the mustard with the orange juice and vinegar. Add the oils, pouring in a slow steady stream. Add the zest, tarragon, and salt and pepper to taste. Set aside.

2. Mix the beet dice with the rice. Add the Jerusalem artichoke and green beans. Moisten with 2 tablespoons of the vinaigrette. Add salt and pepper to taste. Add half of the orange to the rice mixture.

3. Place the greens on a plate. Top with the rice beet mixture, and garnish with the remaining orange sections. Serve the vinaigrette on the side.

BLACK BEAN AND RICE SALAD

This simple but luscious salad is a great way to use up the Mexican Rice and Beans leftovers from dinner. You get lots of fiber from the black beans and brown rice—fiber that protects your colon, promotes weight loss, and helps lower cholesterol. The tomatoes, jicama, and red pepper are all Microbiome Superfoods that will help nourish your microbiome. And the mango salsa adds a zingy sweet taste that helps bring the whole dish to life.

1 SERVING

½ cup cooked brown rice

3 tablespoons Orange Cumin Vinaigrette (page 309), divided

½ cup cooked black beans

1 heaping cup mixed greens

¼ fresh mango, peeled, pitted, in ¼-inch slices

¼ avocado, peeled, pitted, in ¼-inch slices

6 cherry tomatoes, halved

1 teaspoon cilantro, chopped

1½-inch-thick slice of jicama, in ¼-inch dice

1 tablespoon diced raw sweet red pepper

¼ cup Mango Salsa (page 306)

1. In separate bowls, mix the brown rice with 1 tablespoon vinaigrette, mix the beans with 1 tablespoon vinaigrette, and mix the greens with ½ tablespoon vinaigrette. Lay a bed of greens on a dinner plate. Place the rice and the beans on the greens. Surround the rice and beans with the mango, avocado, and tomatoes. Sprinkle the cilantro, jicama, and red pepper on top.

2. Drizzle the remaining vinaigrette on the salad. Serve with the Mango Salsa on the side.

CHÈVRE, BEETS, AND JICAMA SALAD

PHASE 2

Earthy beets, creamy chèvre, piquant arugula, crunchy jicama, and savory herbs are a perfect combination of taste, texture, and aroma. If you're feeling creative and can find them in your produce section, edible nasturtium flowers add a peppery and colorful garnish.

Jicama is a Microbiome Superfood, and the greens load you up with stamina-building iron and B vitamins, which help you to balance your hormones and cope with stress.

2 SERVINGS

1 teaspoon each: fresh tarragon, thyme, chive, and
   parsley, stemmed and snipped

⅛ cup olive oil

½ cup creamy chèvre, preferably Rawson Brook
   Farm's Monterey Chèvre

3 cups mixed greens

1 cup baby arugula or watercress

¼ cup peeled, diced jicama

3 tablespoons Lemon Vinaigrette (see page 263)

2 cooked beets, peeled, quartered, and sliced

Stems of fresh herbs for garnish

2 nasturtium blossoms for garnish (optional)

1. Mix the herbs with the oil. Divide the chèvre into 2 scoops, and pour the herbed oil over them.

2. In a bowl, mix the greens, arugula, and jicama, and toss with the Lemon Vinaigrette.

3. Place the mixture in a shallow bowl, and top with the chèvre scoops.

4. Garnish with the beets and stems of fresh herbs. Top with optional nasturtium blossoms.

Chicken Salad with Fennel, Tomato, Olives, Jicama, and Greens

Looking for a great way to use up leftover chicken? This chicken salad features the Microbiome Superfoods radishes and jicama, which will nourish your microbiome. Enjoy the amazing antioxidant and anti-inflammatory benefits from the fennel and the healthy serving of fiber in the fennel and mixed greens.

1 SERVING

1 heaping cup mixed greens

2 radishes, in ¼-inch slices

4 ¼-inch slices fennel

2 tablespoons Lemon Vinaigrette (page 263), divided

1 cooked chicken breast or meat from 1 leg, sliced

6 cherry tomatoes, halved

6 olives

1 ¼-inch slice jicama, diced

¼ avocado, sliced (optional)

1 tablespoon walnuts or almonds (optional)

1. Mix the greens, radishes, and fennel with 1 tablespoon of the vinaigrette.

2. Place the mixture on a dinner plate, and top with the chicken and remaining ingredients.

3. Drizzle with remaining vinaigrette and serve.

CHICKEN SOUP WITH KALE
AND JERUSALEM ARTICHOKES

PHASE 1

Rich chicken soup is enhanced with Jerusalem artichokes and flavored with garlic to help heal your digestive tract. Kale is a dark green leafy vegetable that boosts your supply of iron, which builds energy through red blood cells, and vitamin B, which you need to modulate stress, support your brain, and balance your hormones. If you have made Chicken Base (page 289) ahead of time and frozen it, putting this soup together goes very quickly.

4 SERVINGS

Juice from ½ lemon, approximately 1 teaspoon

1 cup cold water

3 medium Jerusalem artichokes

1 tablespoon olive oil

1 teaspoon chopped garlic

1 pound fresh kale, ribs removed, washed, still wet

4 cups Chicken Base (page 289)

1 cup chicken pieces (optional)

Salt and pepper to taste

1. Add lemon juice to the cold water in a medium bowl. Scrub Jerusalem artichokes, and cut into ¼-inch slices. Let them soak in the lemon water and set aside.

2. Warm olive oil in a sauté pan over very low heat and add the garlic. Don't let the garlic brown—just leave it in the oil for about 2 minutes. Then add the wet kale and simmer gently, until tender, about 8 minutes.

3. Melt the frozen Chicken Base in a saucepan. Drain the Jerusalem artichokes, and add them to the Chicken Base. Simmer for 10 minutes until tender. Add the kale mixture. Add chicken, if desired. Cook for 10 minutes or until the vegetables are tender. Salt and pepper to taste.

CLASSIC GREEK SALAD WITH
SHEEP'S MILK FETA

This is a quick and easy way to prepare a class Greek salad. Enjoy the fresh, tasty ingredients, which include the Microbiome Superfoods tomato, red pepper, and onions. Nourish your microbiome while you refresh your palate and perk up your lunch hour.

1 SERVING

2 cups romaine lettuce, torn into 1-inch pieces

1 medium tomato, cut into ½-inch chunks

8 Greek olives (kalamata)

¼ peeled cucumber, cut into ½-inch chunks

¼ sweet red pepper, cut into ½-inch chunks

¼ green pepper, cut into ½-inch chunks

2 thin slices red onion (optional)

⅛ teaspoon dried oregano

2 tablespoons Lemon Vinaigrette (page 263)

Salt and pepper to taste

⅛ cup crumbled sheep's milk feta cheese

¼ lemon

1. In a medium bowl, mix together the lettuce, tomato, olives, cucumber, red and green peppers, and onion, if desired.

2. In a separate bowl, mix the oregano into the vinaigrette, and shake vigorously. Add salt and pepper to taste.

3. Place the vegetable mixture on a dinner plate, and top with feta crumbles.

4. Serve with the vinaigrette and a wedge of lemon.

Escarole Chickpea Soup

The rich bone broth in the chicken base make this a supernutritious and hearty soup, and the escarole adds stamina-building iron and B vitamins that help ward off the effects of stress. Onions, garlic, and tomato add three Microbiome Superfoods, while the chickpeas help women balance their hormones, especially during perimenopause and menopause. Sriracha, by the way, is a kind of Thai hot sauce that can give this fragrant soup an extra kick.

3 SERVINGS

1 teaspoon chopped garlic

3 tablespoons olive oil

½ small onion, peeled and chopped

2 cups Chicken Base (see page 289)

4 heaping cups chopped escarole

½ cup organic chickpeas, drained and rinsed

½ cup diced tomatoes

½ teaspoon cumin

1 teaspoon salt

½ cup chopped chicken (optional)

½ teaspoon hot sauce or sriracha (optional)

1. Warm the garlic in a medium saucepan over low heat in the oil, then add the onion. Sauté over medium-low heat until the onion is soft, about 5 minutes.

2. Add the stock and bring to a boil. Add the escarole, chickpeas, and tomatoes. Lower the heat to medium, and simmer for 10 minutes.

3. Add the cumin, salt, and chicken and hot sauce, if desired. Salt to taste.

Fennel Salad

If you're looking for a healthy salad that is also filling, you can't do better than fennel. Crunchy and slightly sweet, this Italian vegetable tastes delicious cooked or raw. You'll get lots of digestive and weight-loss benefits from the fiber, as well as lots of potassium, vitamin C, copper, and manganese. These ingredients also support your immune and cardiovascular systems. Come for the health and weight loss—stay for the refreshing taste!

1 SERVING

½ fennel bulb, stalks removed, thinly sliced crosswise

1 tablespoon olive oil

½ teaspoon fresh lemon juice

½ teaspoon snipped fresh tarragon

Salt and pepper to taste

1. Toss all ingredients together, and serve.

PHASE 1

GUACAMOLE SMOOTHIE

This smoothie is an incredibly rich and creamy pick-me-up. Flaxseed oil adds beneficial Omega 3s, the avocado provides even more healthy fats, the lime juice adds zing, and the pea protein powder gives you a much-needed protein boost to keep you going in the middle of the day. This smoothie is good for a satisfying snack or quick but filling lunch. Olé!

1 SERVING

1 small ripe avocado, peeled and seeded, about ½ cup

2 tablespoons sweet red onion, chopped

¼ cup chopped tomato

¼ teaspoon ground cumin

¼ teaspoon chopped garlic

¼ teaspoon chopped jalapeño pepper or ½ teaspoon
   hot sauce

1 teaspoon olive oil

1 teaspoon flaxseed oil

1 teaspoon fresh lime juice

2 tablespoons pea protein powder

½ teaspoon salt

½ cup water

3 ice cubes

1. Blend all ingredients in a food processor until smooth.

KALE SALAD À LA GREQUE

Kale is loaded with iron, which supports your production of energizing red blood cells, and B vitamins, which are great for combating stress, supporting brain function, and balancing your hormones. The olive oil and olives provide healthy fat to feed your cells and support your brain. The optional chickpeas add protein, make the salad more filling, and help women balance their hormones, especially during perimenopause and just after menopause. The optional quinoa adds still more protein and makes the salad even more filling.

1 SERVING

2 cups kale greens, washed and dried, ribs removed, and
    sliced into thin ribbons

1 teaspoon olive oil

¼ teaspoon salt

2 teaspoons Dijon mustard

2 tablespoons fresh lemon juice

2 tablespoons cider vinegar

⅓ cup olive oil

¼ teaspoon lemon zest, finely chopped (be sure to use
    only the yellow rind, not the white pulp)

Salt and cracked pepper to taste

½ cup canned organic chickpeas, drained and rinsed
    (optional)

¼ avocado, sliced (optional)

3 thin slices red onion (optional)

½ cup cooked quinoa (optional)

½ tomato, chopped, or 6 cherry tomatoes

⅓ cucumber, seeded and chopped

⅓ sweet red pepper, chopped

2 tablespoons chopped Jerusalem artichokes or jicama

8 kalamata olives

¼ cup sheep's milk feta cheese

1. Put the kale in a bowl. Add olive oil and salt. Toss the kale with your hands until it is well coated. Set aside.

2. In a bowl, combine the mustard with the lemon juice and vinegar. Whisk until smooth, and slowly add the olive oil in a slow, steady stream. Add lemon zest, salt, and pepper to taste.

3. Add some of the dressing to the kale. Add the remaining ingredients and toss. Season with salt and pepper to taste.

LEEK, ONION, AND POTATO SOUP   PHASE 2

This creamy soup brings the traditional flavors of France to your lunch table while loading you up with two Microbiome Superfoods—leeks and onions. It will keep in the fridge for two or three days, but don't try freezing it—potatoes don't freeze well. Make it with the Chicken or Beef Base you prepared ahead of time (pages 289 and 278). You can substitute canned or boxed organic beef stock if you prefer, but please make the Chicken Base from scratch—you want to load up on all the healing nutrients from that bone broth, which you will never find in a commercial preparation.

2 SERVINGS

2 large leeks, cleaned and sliced

2 cups sliced onions

1 tablespoon olive oil

2 teaspoons salt

½ teaspoon pepper

2 tablespoons clarified butter

1½ tablespoons gluten-free flour

2 cups Chicken Base (see page 289)

2 cups Beef Base (see page 278)

2 cups peeled, diced potatoes

2 teaspoons dried tarragon

Salt and pepper to taste

1 tablespoon snipped fresh chives or 1 tablespoon
   snipped fresh tarragon

1. Sauté leeks and onion in olive oil in a 12-inch sauté pan over medium-low heat for 10 minutes. Sprinkle with salt and pepper.

2. Add the clarified butter, and, when melted, stir in the flour. Cook on low for 2 minutes. Stir in the stocks, and whisk for 1 minute.

3. Add the potatoes and dried tarragon. Bring to a simmer, and cook for 40 minutes or until potatoes are tender. Let cool.

4. Puree the soup in a blender or use an immersion blender.

5. Salt and pepper to taste. Garnish with snipped chives.

MANGO ARUGULA SALAD

This sweet, piquant salad will leave you both refreshed and satisfied. The mango is full of vitamins A and C, which help repair your gut walls and support your immune system, jicama and tomato nourish your microbiome, and the avocado loads you up with healthy fats. Find directions for peeling the mango on page 255. Find the recipe for Citrus Vinaigrette on page 261. If you're taking this to work, don't add the last of the dressing at home; instead, take it to work with you in a small jar and drizzle it on just before you eat.

1 SERVING

2 cups arugula leaves

2 tablespoons Citrus Vinaigrette (page 261)

½ small avocado, peeled and sliced

½ small mango, peeled and cut into slices

¼ red onion, thinly sliced

Salt and pepper to taste

Chicken slices (optional)

1. Toss the arugula leaves with half of the vinaigrette.

2. Add the avocado, mango, and onion to the arugula mix, and salt and pepper to taste. Add the chicken if desired.

3. Drizzle the remaining vinaigrette on top. Serve immediately.

PREBIOTIC SUPERFOOD GREEN SALAD WITH LEMON VINAIGRETTE

 PHASE 1

There's nothing like a fresh green salad loaded with vibrant vegetables to leave you feeling refreshed and energized in the middle of the day. This healthy salad is loaded with prebiotics to nourish your microbiome.

1 SERVING

2 cups mixed-lettuce greens

¼ fennel bulb, sliced into ¼-inch slices

1 small tomato, cut into ¼-inch slices

1 small Jerusalem artichoke, scrubbed, with hard ends removed, cut into ¼-inch slices

3 radishes, washed, with ends removed, cut into ¼-inch slices

Lemon Vinaigrette (page 263)

1. Combine greens, fennel, tomato, Jerusalem Artichoke, and radishes, and toss with Lemon Vinaigrette.

RICH VEGETABLE SOUP

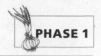
PHASE 1

The French call this type of soup "Soupe a la pistou": a fragrant vegetable soup garnished with *pistou*, a savory infusion of chopped fresh basil, garlic, and tomato. It's a wonderful way to load up on vegetables, which will leave you feeling full and satisfied without that overstuffed, bloated feeling you can sometimes get from too much meat or starch. You're also loading up on Microbiome Superfoods—leeks and carrots in the soup and garlic and tomato in the pistou. If you're looking for some extra protein, add the chicken pieces. The pistou makes enough for a few servings and will keep well in the fridge or freezer.

3 SERVINGS

2 tablespoons olive oil

1 leek, washed and sliced, green tops discarded

¼ bunch kale, washed, ribs removed, rough chopped

1 tablespoon chopped garlic

1 small turnip, peeled and chopped

1 celery stalk, chopped

1 carrot, peeled and chopped

1 parsnip, peeled and sliced

3 cups Chicken Base (page 289)

1 zucchini, diced

¼ pound mushrooms, stemmed, cleaned, and sliced

¼ cup cooked chicken pieces (optional)

PISTOU

2 tablespoons minced garlic

4 cups basil leaves (about 2 ounces)

⅓ cup rough chopped tomatoes or 3 tablespoons organic tomato paste

½ teaspoon salt

½ teaspoon pepper

⅓ cup olive oil

Salt and pepper

1. In a large, heavy-bottomed pot, gently heat olive oil over medium-low heat, add leek and kale, and cook 5 minutes until golden. Add garlic, and cook for 2 minutes.

2. Add the turnip, celery, carrot, and parsnip, and cook for 5 minutes. Add the Chicken Base, and simmer for 45 minutes or until vegetables are tender.

3. Add the zucchini, mushrooms, and optional chicken, and simmer for 10 minutes until tender.

4. Make the pistou: while the soup is cooking, put the garlic, basil, tomatoes, and salt and pepper in a food processor or blender, and puree until almost smooth. Gradually add the oil. Refrigerate until ready to serve.

5. To serve, stir 3 tablespoons of the pistou into the hot soup. Add salt, pepper, and more pistou to taste.

RUMANIAN EGGPLANT SALAD PHASE 1

You might be more familiar with eggplant that has been breaded and fried, but in this salad you simply pan-sear it, which brings out its rich, earthy taste, enhanced by the tangy vinegar and lemon. When you choose an eggplant, make sure it is shiny, light, and firm with no soft spots. You can enhance the flavor of the chopped, seasoned eggplant by refrigerating it for a few days. For one serving, simply prepare one-third the amount of each vegetable.

3 SERVINGS

1 large, firm eggplant

1 tablespoon cider vinegar

1 tablespoon salt

3 tablespoons olive oil

4 cups mixed greens

21 cherry tomatoes or 4 small tomatoes, sliced

1 bulb fennel, thinly sliced

4 small Jerusalem artichokes, thinly sliced or ½ medium
    jicama, thinly sliced

1 medium cucumber, peeled and seeded, sliced

Salt and pepper to taste

Lemon Vinaigrette, approximately 4 teaspoons (see
  page 263)

1. Wrap the firm eggplant in heavy aluminum foil. Heat a cast-iron skillet, and place the eggplant in the skillet. Turn heat up to medium-high, and cook the eggplant, turning every 5 minutes until it is collapsed. Let cool, unwrap, and scoop the soft, well-cooked eggplant from the skin.

2. Place the eggplant flesh in a food processor, and process for 15 seconds. Add the vinegar and salt, and pulse, adding the oil in slow stream. As soon as the oil is incorporated, stop processing so the eggplant is not pureed.

3. Place the eggplant on the greens, and surround with the tomato, fennel, Jerusalem artichokes, and cucumber. Salt and pepper to taste. Drizzle vinaigrette on the sliced vegetables.

SAUERKRAUT AND MEATBALL SOUP 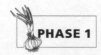 PHASE 1

This hearty entrée soup for lunch or dinner was inspired by Eastern European–style stuffed cabbage. It's warm and filling, and because it contains sauerkraut, a fermented food, it is also a natural probiotic. Plus it contains several Microbiome Superfoods—onions, garlic, carrots, and the Microbiome Superspice, cinnamon.

Save five of the meatballs to serve with Roasted Spaghetti Squash (page 304). Buy the sauerkraut in the fermented foods section of the market. The beef stock takes 5 hours to cook, but you can make it ahead of time or just substitute canned or boxed organic beef stock. The soup freezes very well.

6 SERVINGS, PLUS 4 CUPS STOCK TO BE FROZEN

BEEF BASE

3 pounds beef shin bone

2 marrow bones

1 pound beef chuck, cut in thirds

3 quarts water

1 unpeeled onion, studded with 6 cloves

1 carrot washed and trimmed, cut into ¾-inch pieces

3 sprigs parsley

3 peppercorns

FOR THE MEATBALLS

½ cup chopped onion

1½ pounds ground beef

1 small egg

½ teaspoon freshly ground nutmeg

1 tablespoon kosher salt

½ teaspoon freshly ground pepper

FOR THE SOUP

2 tablespoons olive oil

2 onions, sliced

2 carrots, peeled and sliced

2 parsnips, peeled and sliced

5 cups Beef Base

1 28-ounce can organic chopped tomatoes

¼ cup cider vinegar

10 whole cloves

1 teaspoon cinnamon

1 teaspoon ground nutmeg

1 teaspoon ground allspice

3 teaspoons sugar substitute: Lakanta

2 cups sauerkraut, drained

To make the Beef Base

1. In a large pot, cook the beef and marrow bones in boiling water for five minutes. Drain, discarding the water.

2. Place the bones back into the pot, and add the beef chuck and 3 quarts of water. Bring to a boil, and then reduce the heat. Skim off the fat and foam until it stops forming, about 15 minutes.

3. Add the onion, carrot, parsley, peppercorns, and salt. Simmer 3 hours.

4. Strain the liquid and taste for seasoning. If the flavor is not concentrated enough, continue cooking over medium heat until the desired taste is achieved. If you like, add more salt to taste. This will yield almost 3 quarts of stock. Strain the stock and refrigerate so the fat solidifies and can be easily removed. When chilled, skim the fat off the top, and discard. Use 5 cups of the stock for the recipe, and freeze the remainder.

For the meatballs and soup

1. Preheat oven to 375°F. Lightly oil a 12 x 18-inch sheet pan.

2. For the meatballs, sauté the chopped onion until it is golden, and set aside.

3. For the soup, in oil, lightly sauté the sliced onion, carrots, and parsnips over medium heat for 10 minutes, until vegetables are tender. Remove from pan, and set aside.

4. To make the meatballs, combine the ground beef, sautéed onion, egg, nutmeg, salt, and pepper in a medium bowl. Form into 1½-inch-size meatballs, and place on an oiled baking sheet. Place in a preheated 375°F oven for 30 minutes. Let cool and set aside.

5. While the meatballs are cooking, heat the stock over medium flame. Add the vegetable mixture, and simmer about 10 minutes.

6. Add the tomatoes, vinegar, cloves, cinnamon, nutmeg, allspice, and Lakanta. Stir and cook for 10 minutes. Add the sauerkraut, cook for 5 minutes, and taste for seasoning.

7. Before serving, add the meatballs, and cook over medium heat for 5 minutes. Salt and pepper to taste.

PHASE 2

SAVORY PEAR SALAD

This was a favorite at Chef Carole's restaurant, Charleston. Pears, walnuts, and blue cheese are a luscious combination. The walnuts and vinaigrette provide healthy fats for your cells and brain, and the mixed greens are rich in energizing iron and stress-busting B vitamins.

2 SERVINGS

1 large or 2 small ripe pears

4 cups mixed greens

⅓ cup crumbled sheep's or goat's milk blue cheese

¼ cup broken walnut halves

3 tablespoons Citrus Vinaigrette (page 261)

Salt and pepper to taste

5 slices cooked cold chicken breast

1. Halve, quarter and slice the pears. Set six slices aside for garnish.

2. Arrange the greens in a shallow bowl. Add the pear, cheese, and walnuts. Toss with the vinaigrette. Add salt and pepper to taste.

3. Mound the greens and garnish with the set aside pear slices, sliced chicken, and any additional walnuts.

TURKISH-STYLE CUCUMBER SOUP   PHASE 2

This cold soup makes a refreshing lunch or snack. The live cultures in the yogurt give your microbiome a major boost, while the protein supports your energy. Cool and tangy, the aromatic flavors of mint and dill make the soup extra flavorful, and the garnishes of tomato and Jerusalem artichoke give you two helpings of Microbiome Superfoods. If you want to make the soup more filling, throw in the optional quinoa. Anything left over will keep for a few days in the fridge.

2 SERVINGS

1 large cucumber, peeled and seeded

1½ cups goat's or sheep's milk yogurt

1½ teaspoons minced garlic

1 tablespoon cold water

½ teaspoon salt

½ teaspoon pepper

1 teaspoon white vinegar

1 tablespoon olive oil

¼ cup and 1 tablespoon chopped fresh mint

¼ cup and one tablespoon chopped fresh dill

½ cup cooked quinoa (optional)

FOR GARNISH

2 tablespoons chopped fresh tomato

2 tablespoons diced Jerusalem artichoke or jicama

Fresh dill

Fresh mint

1. Dice ¼ cup of the cucumber for garnish and set aside. Grate the remainder.

2. Combine the yogurt, garlic, water, salt, pepper, vinegar, olive oil, and ¼ cup of each herb in a medium-large bowl. Add the quinoa if desired.

3. Add the shredded cucumber. Refrigerate for 3 hours or more.

4. When ready to serve, taste for seasoning and add more salt and pepper. Garnish with the chopped tomato, Jerusalem artichoke, dill, and mint.

DINNERS

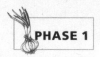

PHASE 1

BASIL PESTO

This delicious Italian dish is a wonderful way to enjoy the green taste of fresh basil, enlivened with the zingy flavors of lemon and garlic. Pesto is traditionally served on pasta, so it will go beautifully with our Microbiome Diet recipe for "spaghetti squash." I've had you make some extra; refrigerate it in an airtight container, and you can continue to use the leftovers as a vegetable dip. Make sure you find fresh basil—the recipe definitely will not work with dried.

1 CUP

2 heaping cups fresh basil leaves

2 garlic cloves, peeled and sliced

⅓ cup pine nuts

½ cup olive oil

¼ cup sunflower oil

1 tablespoon freshly squeezed lemon juice

1 teaspoon salt

1. Place all the ingredients in a food processor, and process until smooth.
2. Refrigerate remaining pesto for future use.

BEEF, BEER, AND ONION STEW

This Belgian-style beef stew, *Carbonnades a la Flammande*, is rich, hearty, and satisfying. The beer—gluten-free and Belgian style—gives a rich, hearty taste to the meat, while the onions add a touch of sweetness.

This recipe can be made ahead of time and then refrigerated for four days. It also freezes well. Reheat the defrosted stew in a preheated 350°F oven.

3 SERVINGS

1½ pounds stewing beef, cut in 1-inch pieces

1 tablespoon rice flour

1 teaspoon salt

½ teaspoon pepper

1 tablespoon olive oil

4 cups sliced onions

2 garlic cloves, minced

1 teaspoon salt

½ teaspoon pepper

1½ cups gluten-free beer, divided

½ cup strong organic Beef Base (see page 278)

3 tablespoons Lakanto, a sugar substitute, divided

1 teaspoon dried thyme

2 tablespoons cider vinegar

Salt and pepper to taste

1. Preheat oven to 350°F.

2. Dry the beef with paper towels. On a 9-inch plate, mix together the beef, rice flour, salt, and pepper until the beef is well coated. Reserve leftover rice flour mixture.

3. Heat the oil in a 9- or 10-inch fireproof Dutch oven casserole; add the meat. Over medium-high heat brown the meat on all sides, which takes approximately 5 minutes. Remove the meat. Add the onions to the pot and cook, stirring con-tinually for 5 minutes. Add salt, pepper, garlic and 1 teaspoon of the leftover rice flour mixture.

4. After about 5 minutes, the onion mixture should be light brown. Then add ½ cup of the beer, and scrape up the browned bits on the bottom of the pot. Add the beef, and stir in the remaining beer, Beef Base, 1 tablespoon Lakanto, and thyme.

5. Bring to a simmer, and then reduce the heat to low. Cover the casserole, and cook at 350°F for about 2 hours; testing the beef for tenderness—cook until the meat is fork tender. Add the vinegar and 2 remaining tablespoons Lakanto, and cook for 3 minutes longer. Taste for seasoning, adding salt and pepper and more thyme to taste.

BEEF STEW WITH AROMATIC VEGETABLES AND RED WINE

PHASE 1

Here's another hearty stew, this time with a French influence. The ar-omatic vegetables add a delicate flavor to the mix, while the red wine brings out all the flavor of the beef. You also get plenty of onions and carrots in this dish, two Microbiome Superfoods.

This stew can be cooked in advanced and kept refrigerated for up to four days. Or you can freeze it and keep it for weeks. To reheat, bring to room temperature and then cook for approximately ten minutes on low heat.

2 SERVINGS

¾ cup chopped onions

⅓ cup chopped carrots

1 large garlic clove, minced

⅓ cup chopped parsnips

1 tablespoon coconut oil

1 tablespoon rice flour

1 teaspoon salt

½ teaspoon pepper

½ teaspoon grated nutmeg

1 pound stew beef, cut into 2-inch pieces

1 cup Beef or Chicken Base (see pages 278 and 289, respectively), divided

½ teaspoon thyme

1 spray rosemary

1 teaspoon tarragon

1 cup red wine

1 onion, peeled and sliced

2 tablespoons clarified butter or olive oil, divided

⅓ pound mushrooms, sliced

Chopped parsley for garnish

1. Preheat oven to 300°F.

2. In a large ovenproof, lidded pot, sauté the chopped onion, carrot, garlic, and parsnips in the coconut oil over medium-low heat for 8 minutes until vegetables are tender. Remove from the pan and set aside.

3. In a medium bowl, combine the rice flour, salt, pepper, nutmeg, and beef. The beef should be well coated with flour mixture.

4. Add more oil to the pot if necessary, and transfer the meat to the pot, sautéing over medium-high heat until the meat is browned, about 8 minutes. Remove the meat, and add ½ cup of the Beef Base to the pot to scrape up the browned bits.

5. Transfer the vegetable mixture and the meat back to the pot. Add the thyme, rosemary, tarragon, red wine, and remaining stock. Bring to a boil, lower the heat, and place in oven, cooking at 300°F for about 2 hours; after 1½ hours check for tenderness.

6. While the stew is cooking, sauté the sliced onions in 1 tablespoon of the butter. Remove from pan. Sauté the mushrooms in remaining butter. Add mushrooms to onions and set aside.

7. Add the onion and mushroom mixture to the stew ½ hour before serving.

8. Add salt and pepper for taste. Garnish with chopped parsley.

BORSCHT

Ah, Mother Russia! This robust lunch or dinner entrée soup will charm you with its sweet and sour flavors while leaving you feeling full and satisfied from its rich, meaty broth. Add in some white beans to make the dish even more filling.

To make this dish you'll need the Beef Base you prepared ahead of time, or you can just use canned or boxed organic beef stock. (But the homemade will taste better!) Enjoy the flavors while knowing you are loading up on Microbiome Superfoods: onion, carrot, tomato, and garlic.

6 TO 8 SERVINGS

6 medium beets, scrubbed

2 medium onions, chopped

4 carrots, peeled and grated

3 tablespoons olive oil

2 pounds boneless stew beef, cut into 1-inch cubes

3 tablespoons organic tomato paste

6 to 8 cups Beef Base (see page 278), divided

12 whole garlic cloves

6 peppercorns

2 tablespoons Lakanto

1 tablespoon cider vinegar

½ head cabbage, shredded

1 tablespoon chopped fresh dill

4 teaspoons salt

1 teaspoon pepper

1. In a large saucepan, boil the beets for about 45 minutes, until they can be pierced with a butter knife. Remove from heat, and allow to cool, saving the beet water. Slip the skins off the beets, and discard. Cut the beets into match sticks.

2. In a medium pan over medium heat, sauté onions and carrots in the oil, about 5 minutes. Add the beef, and cook until brown, about 10 minutes. Add the tomato paste and a cup of the stock. Set aside.

3. Combine the remaining stock, 1 to 2 cups beet water, beef mixture, garlic, peppercorns, and beets in a large pot. Add the Lakanto and vinegar. Cook 20 minutes over low heat. Add the cabbage, and cook until the cabbage is tender, about 10 minutes. Add dill, as well as more Lakanto, salt, and pepper to taste. The soup should have a sweet and sour flavor.

BRAISED APPLE CHICKEN

This supper can easily be made ahead and either refrigerated or frozen. The sweetness of the apples and cider make the chicken taste sweet as well, while the coconut oil adds a serving of healthy fat. The apples are full of fiber that nourishes your microbiome.

When you are shopping for this dinner choose apples that are firm and not bruised.

2 SERVINGS

2 skinless, boneless chicken breasts or thighs

Salt and pepper to taste

2 tablespoons coconut oil, divided

1 cup unsweetened apple cider, divided

2 cups peeled, sliced onions

2 cups peeled, cored, seeded, and sliced apples

1 tablespoon dried tarragon

½ teaspoon dried thyme

½ teaspoon salt

¼ teaspoon pepper

1. Preheat oven to 375°F.

2. Sprinkle chicken with salt and pepper. In a small sauté pan, sauté the chicken in 1 tablespoon coconut oil on medium-low heat until lightly browned. Remove from pan, and deglaze pan with ¼ cup of the apple cider, scraping all the browned bits into the cider. Pour this deglazing cider over the chicken, and set aside. Clean the pan.

3. Sauté onions in remaining coconut oil over low heat for 5 minutes, until softened. Add the apples, and cook for 5 minutes.

4. Add the chicken, deglazing liquid, tarragon, thyme, and the remaining cider. Season with salt and pepper.

5. Transfer to a small ovenproof baking pan, cover with a lid or foil, and bake at 375°F for 20 minutes. Turn chicken over, and bake uncovered for an additional 10 minutes or until the chicken is no longer pink and the juices are clear.

6. Add salt and pepper to taste if desired.

Brazilian Fish Stew

Maybe you don't have time to fly down to Carnival in Rio this year, but you definitely do have time to make this quick and easy Brazilian-flavored coconut-creamy stew. Delicious with any firm-fleshed fish, the stew works with cod, grouper, catfish, and similar choices. Just make sure you go low mercury.

For added digestive healing—and creamy sweetness—enjoy the coconut milk. Garlic, onion, and tomato will help heal your intestinal tract while nourishing your microbiome.

2 SERVINGS

1 pound cod, or any firm fish

2 tablespoons lime juice

1 garlic clove, finely chopped

½ teaspoon salt

¼ teaspoon pepper

½ cup chopped onion

1 teaspoon paprika

⅓ cup diced red pepper

1 tablespoon coconut oil

½ cup diced tomato

½ cup coconut milk

½ teaspoon hot sauce, or more to taste

½ cup chopped cilantro, divided

1. Place the fish in a small bowl, and cover with the lime juice, garlic, salt, and pepper. Marinate for 15 minutes.

2. Sauté the onion, paprika, and red pepper in the coconut oil on medium-low for 5 minutes until soft. Add the tomato and marinated fish, and cook until the fish begins to turn opaque, about 5 minutes.

3. Add the coconut milk, hot sauce, and half of the cilantro. Simmer until the fish is fully opaque and begins to flake, about 10 to 15 minutes. Taste for seasoning. Add more lime juice, hot sauce, and salt to taste.

4. Add the remaining cilantro and serve.

CHICKEN BASE

How healthy can you get—not just the chicken, but the bones as well, which are liquefied and strained into the soup. This "bone broth" heals and seals the gut wall and is loaded with minerals. The broth requires many hours for simmering, but once you've made it, you can divide it into 2-cup containers and freeze enough portions to last you a few weeks. Use it as your base for the traditional chicken soup as well as for the vegetable soups and sauces.

10 CUPS

1 5- to 6-pound chicken, cut up, rinsed, and dried

2 garlic cloves, finely chopped

3 tablespoons salt, or more to taste

16 cups cold water

2 large onions, quartered, unpeeled

1 large carrot, cut into 4 pieces, unpeeled

5 stems each of parsley and dill, tied in a bunch

½ teaspoon pepper

1. Rub the chicken parts with the garlic and salt; cover and refrigerate 1 hour.

2. Put the water, onions, carrot, and all the chicken parts, except the breasts, into a stockpot. Bring to a boil, and add the breasts and the bunch of parsley and dill. Cover the pot, reduce heat, and simmer for 40 minutes, until tender.

3. Remove the breasts. Skim off fat; discard. Remove the skin and chicken from the breast bones; discard skin. Put the bones back into the pot, and continue cooking for 2 hours. Cut up the chicken into bite-size pieces, and refrigerate or freeze for another use.

4. When tender, remove the remaining chicken from the pot, and continue cooking the bones and stock 30 minutes. Remove the chicken meat from the legs and back. Return the bones to the stock pot, and continue cooking on low heat for 3 hours. Refrigerate or freeze the chicken meat for another use.

5. Remove and discard the vegetables and herbs from the pot. Put the bones and 1 cup of the broth in a blender, and process until liquefied and smooth. Strain the liquid, discard any solids, and strain the liquefied bones back into the stock. Add the pepper, and taste to see if you want to add more salt. There will be about 10 cups of soup base.

6. Refrigerate what you will need for making a soup, and freeze the remainder.

PHASE 2

CHILI CON CARNE

This is a quick and easy chili that freezes well. Or you can store it in an airtight container and keep it in the fridge for up to three days. Onions, garlic, and tomato give you plenty of Microbiome Superfoods to make this dish both superfast *and* superhealthy.

3 SERVINGS

1 medium yellow onion, chopped, about 1 scant cup

2 tablespoons olive oil

1 pound lean ground beef

1 teaspoon chopped jalapeño

2 garlic cloves, minced

½ teaspoon ground oregano

1 tablespoon chili powder

1 tablespoon cumin

1 tablespoon paprika

1 teaspoon salt

½ teaspoon cayenne pepper (optional)

1½ cups organic fire-roasted canned diced tomatoes

½ cup water

1 15-ounce can of organic kidney beans, drained
    and rinsed

Salt and pepper to taste

1. Sauté onion in the oil, cooking for 3 to 4 minutes. Add ground beef, and cook, stirring until beef is no longer pink. With a wooden spoon break up the beef as it cooks.

2. Add the jalapeño, garlic, and spices. Stir and cook for 2 minutes. Stir in the diced tomatoes, water, and kidney beans. Bring to a boil. Lower heat, and simmer for 35 minutes. Add additional salt and pepper to taste.

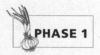

CURRIED LAMB AND LENTIL STEW

Lentils are such a healthy food! They load you up with protein, support your digestion, and leave you feeling full and satisfied. Full of fiber, they are one of your microbiome's favorite foods too.

This quick and easy stew also contains the Microbiome Superspice turmeric, which is a terrific anti-inflammatory that promotes digestive health and supports a healthy brain. The coconut milk provides you with some healthy fat and a sweet, creamy flavor that compliments the taste of the lamb.

2 SERVINGS

½ boneless stew lamb, cut into 1-inch pieces

1 teaspoon salt

½ teaspoon pepper

1 tablespoon olive oil

½ heaping cup chopped onions

½ cup chopped carrots

2 teaspoons chopped garlic

1 tablespoon finely chopped fresh ginger

¼ teaspoon turmeric

¼ teaspoon cumin

1 tablespoon curry powder

1 teaspoon kosher salt

¾ cup diced tomatoes

½ cup dried lentils

1 large carrot, cut into coins

¼ cup coconut milk

¼ cup water

1. Sprinkle lamb with salt and pepper.

2. Heat oil in a heavy pan over medium-high heat, and sauté lamb until brown, about 7 to 8 minutes. Add onions, carrots, garlic, and ginger. Mix and sauté on low heat for 3 to 4 minutes. Add turmeric, cumin, curry, and salt, and stir. Add tomatoes, lentils, carrots, coconut milk, and water. Bring to boil, lower heat, and cook until lamb and lentils are tender, about 45 minutes.

CURRIED VEGETABLE STEW

This sumptuous vegetarian dinner is packed with nutrient-rich vegetables as well as chickpeas, which help women balance their hormones, and coconut milk, which adds healthy fats that support your cell and brain health.

The creamy curry sauce really sets off all the different textures of the fresh vegetables. The chickpeas and the optional butternut squash make this a very satisfying meal that will leave you feeling full and nourished but not stuffed. This stew will keep for up to a week or so in the fridge, so once it's made you can enjoy it for several days.

3 SERVINGS

1 cup sliced carrots

2 cups cauliflower florets

1 large onion, sliced

2 tablespoons clarified butter or olive oil

1 tablespoon minced garlic

1 teaspoon finely chopped jalapeño pepper

1 tablespoon chopped fresh ginger

½ teaspoon turmeric

2 tablespoons curry powder

¼ small cabbage, sliced

1 cup diced butternut squash (optional)

½ cup green peas

1½ cups coconut milk

½ cup organic chickpeas

Salt and pepper to taste

¼ cup chopped cilantro

1. In a medium pot, boil 3 cups of water. Place the carrots and cauliflower in a strainer basket in the boiling water for 5 minutes, then remove from the heat.

2. Sauté the onion in clarified butter until softened, about 5 minutes. Add the garlic, jalapeño, ginger, turmeric, and curry. Stir to combine, and cook on low heat for 3 minutes. Add the cabbage, squash, peas, carrots, and cauliflower, and cook gently for 2 minutes, stirring to combine well.

3. Add the coconut milk and chickpeas, and cook for about 20 minutes, until the cauliflower is tender. Add more coconut milk if necessary to make sure the stew is saucy.

4. Taste for seasoning, and add salt, pepper, and more jalapeño to taste. To serve, sprinkle with the chopped cilantro.

Easy Sautéed Greens

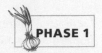
PHASE 1

Looking for a quick, easy, and tasty way to get more greens into your diet? Leafy green vegetables are terrific for your health—full of energizing iron, stress-busting B vitamins, and many other valuable nutrients that help heal your gut and support your metabolism.

In this recipe you quickly sauté your greens, wilting them in garlic-scented oil to produce a light, savory vegetable. This recipe can be used with most leafy greens—escarole, spinach, or broccoli rabe. If you happen to find some dandelion greens in the market, you can use this recipe for them as well; just make sure you boil them for 10 minutes before sautéing them. Dandelion greens are a natural prebiotic that also provides you with many other nutrients.

1 SERVING

½ bunch of escarole, spinach, or broccoli rabe

1 tablespoon olive oil

½ teaspoon minced garlic

Salt and pepper

1. Wash the greens, and leave them wet.

2. In a sauté pan, warm olive oil over low heat. Add the greens and garlic; cook over low heat until the greens wilt or until the broccoli rabe florets are tender when pierced with a fork, about 12 minutes. Add salt and pepper to taste.

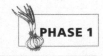
PHASE 1

Fish Stew with Romesco

Bring the flavors of Spain into your kitchen with this riff on a classic Catalan fish stew. The almond garlic infusion is called "romesco," adding a depth of flavor that will leave you feeling satisfied.

This stew can be made with any firm-fleshed white fish—just pick one that is low in mercury, such as catfish, cod, or grouper. The fish and almonds are full of Omega 3 fats, which promote cell and brain health.

For your convenience the romesco recipe yields a cup of sauce, which you can store in the fridge for future use, either to make another stew or as a delicious dip for vegetables.

2 SERVINGS

ROMESCO

1 large tomato

1 cup slivered almonds

½ cup plus 1 tablespoon olive oil, divided

1 teaspoon jalapeño, or more to taste

2 garlic cloves, chopped

½ yellow pepper

2 scallions, trimmed and chopped

1 teaspoon cider vinegar

½ teaspoon salt

1. Preheat oven to 350°F.

2. Place the tomato and the almonds on a baking pan, and bake for 10 minutes, until the almonds start to color. Watch them closely so they don't burn.

3. Add ¼ cup of the oil to a small sauté pan, and sauté the jalapeño over medium heat, about 5 minutes. When the jalapeño is soft, add the garlic. Cook for 2 minutes. Do not allow the garlic to brown. Remove from heat.

4. Put into a food processor the yellow pepper, scallion, and jalapeño mixture.

5. Remove the skin from the tomato, and then add the tomato, vinegar, and almonds to the processor.

6. Process for 1 minute, and slowly add the remaining olive oil. Scrape down the sides of the bowl; add salt, and puree just until smooth.

7. Add more salt to taste, if desired. The sauce can be refrigerated for several days. Serve at room temperature.

FOR THE FISH STEW

¾ cup chopped onion

1 small fennel bulb, sliced

2 tablespoons olive oil

1 garlic clove, minced

½ cup chopped tomatoes

1 cup dry white wine

½ cup bottled clam juice or Chicken Base (see page 289)

1 pound boneless catfish, cod, or grouper cut into 2-inch chunks

Salt and pepper to taste

1. In a sauté pan or small saucepan, sauté the onion and fennel in the olive oil over medium-low heat until tender, for about 8 minutes. Add the garlic and the tomatoes, and cook for 10 minutes. Add the wine and clam juice, and top with the fish; simmer for 8 to 10 minutes until the fish is opaque and cooked.

2. Transfer the fish to serving bowls, and whisk 3 tablespoons Romesco into the soup.

3. Add salt and pepper to taste. Pour the soup over the fish, and serve.

4. Put a dish of Romesco on the table in case you or your dinner companions want more.

GREEK-INSPIRED BEEF STEW WITH ONIONS, FETA CHEESE, AND WALNUTS PHASE 2

This dish was so popular in Chef Carole's restaurant, Charleston, that it inspired the offering of a weekly stew. Not only is it delicious; it's also loaded with Microbiome Superfoods: onions, garlic, and tomatoes plus the Microbiome Superspice, cinnamon. The walnuts add an interesting crunch as well as provide some Omega 3 healthy fats to support cell and brain health.

You can make this stew ahead of time and refrigerate it. It also freezes very well.

SERVES 6

1½ pounds lean beef, cut into 1½-inch cubes

1 tablespoon olive oil

Salt and pepper to taste

2 medium onions, peeled and sliced

1 large garlic clove, minced

¼ cup red wine

1 tablespoon red wine vinegar

2 cups organic diced tomatoes

½ teaspoon ground cinnamon or 1 small cinnamon stick

½ teaspoon freshly ground nutmeg

9 whole cloves

¼ teaspoon ground cumin

½ cup crumbled sheep's milk feta cheese

½ cup walnuts

1. Lightly brown the beef in the olive oil over medium-high heat for 7 to 8 minutes. Add salt and pepper to taste.

2. Cover with the onions, and cook until they begin to soften, about 5 minutes. Add the red wine, wine vinegar, tomatoes, cinnamon, nutmeg, cloves, and cumin. Cover and simmer for 2 hours until the meat is tender. To serve, add the feta cheese and walnuts.

3. Add salt, pepper, and additional feta to taste.

GRILLED BEEF BURGER AND PORTOBELLO MUSHROOM NAPOLEON

You won't miss the hamburger bun at all with this creative combination of burger and Portobello. When buying beef, choose the 80 percent to 20 percent meat-to-fat ratio, as that will provide the juiciest, most tasty burger. The meat should be red, not gray, and preferably freshly ground. Ask your butcher to grind some chuck for you.

When buying the mushrooms, select them from the loose bin. Choose two with firm caps and dry gills. If the gills are black and moist, reject them!

If you don't have a grill, the burgers can be cooked in a black cast-iron pan. Just remember to turn on the exhaust fan!

1 SERVING

8 ounces ground beef

¼ teaspoon of salt, divided

¼ teaspoon pepper, divided

2 Portobello mushrooms, 4 inches in diameter

3 teaspoons olive oil, divided (if using cast-iron skillet)

2 medium slices red onion (optional)

1 heaping cup assorted greens

1 Jerusalem artichoke, scrubbed and thinly sliced

3 thin slices fennel

1 ripe tomato, sliced into 6 to 7 rounds

2 tablespoons Lemon Vinaigrette (see page 263)

Salt and pepper to taste

3 leaves bibb lettuce

¼ avocado, peeled and sliced (optional)

1. In a small bowl, mix the beef with ⅛ teaspoon each of the salt and pepper. With a minimum of handling, form into a 1-inch thick, 4-inch wide patty.

2. Heat the grill to medium high.

3. Remove the stems from the mushrooms, and clean the caps with a dry paper towel or mushroom brush. Brush the mushrooms on both sides with 1 teaspoon of the olive oil, and season with ⅛ teaspoon each of the salt and pepper.

4. Place the mushrooms on the grill, and cook for about 4 to 5 minutes on each side. If you don't have a grill, put a teaspoon of oil in a black cast-iron pan, and cook the mushrooms for about 4 to 5 minutes on each side. The mushrooms will be firm, cooked through, and shrunken in size. Remove and set aside.

5. If using the onions, while the mushrooms are cooking, add the onion to the grill or pan, and cook for 2 minutes until softened. Remove and set aside.

6. Turn up the grill temperature to high heat. If using a cast-iron pan, turn on the exhaust fan, put 1 teaspoon olive oil in the pan, and set heat to medium-high. Cook the burger for 3 to 5 minutes on one side, and then turn for another 3 to 5 minutes on the other side. Do not flatten the burger while cooking, and resist flipping it. When the burger is firm and has a nice crust, remove from the grill to rest.

7. Combine the greens, Jerusalem artichoke, fennel, and all but 3 slices of tomato with the vinaigrette. Salt and pepper to taste.

8. Place one mushroom cap on a plate, and layer with the burger, bibb lettuce, tomato slices, optional avocado, onion, and top with the second mushroom cap. Serve the Burger Napoleon with the salad on the side.

PHASE 2

ITALIAN-ACCENTED CHICKEN STEW

Bring a taste of Italy into your kitchen with this variation on the classic Italian chicken stew, Chicken Cacciatore. Garlic, tomatoes, and onions give you plenty of Microbiome Superfoods, which might be why those ingredients show up so often in traditional Italian cooking.

Ideally you would make this stew on Sunday night and eat it over the next three days, because as the stew sits, the flavors are enhanced. You can also make it ahead of time and freeze it.

2 SERVINGS

Salt and pepper

1 pound boneless chicken breast or thighs

5 tablespoons olive oil, divided

⅓ cup roughly chopped onion

1 large garlic clove, minced

2 tablespoons finely chopped green pepper

1 teaspoon orange zest

1 tablespoon cider vinegar

⅓ cup chicken broth

⅓ cup white vermouth or wine

1 fennel bulb, trimmed and sliced

⅓ cup diced tomatoes or 1 tablespoon tomato paste

2 teaspoons chopped fresh rosemary, divided

2 teaspoons chopped fresh thyme, divided

6 mushrooms, sliced

Salt and pepper

1. Preheat oven to 350°F.

2. Generously salt and pepper the chicken. Brown the chicken in a sauté pan in 3 tablespoons oil over medium-high heat for 10 minutes. Transfer chicken to a baking pan.

3. Add to the sauté pan 2 tablespoons oil along with the onion, garlic, green pepper, and zest, and sauté for 2 minutes. Add the vinegar, broth, vermouth, fennel, tomato, and 1 teaspoon each of the rosemary and thyme, and cook for 3 minutes. Pour the mixture over the chicken, cover the baking pan with foil, place in the oven, and cook at 350°F for 20 minutes.

4. In a medium pan, sauté the mushrooms over medium-low heat for 5 minutes, and sprinkle with the remaining rosemary and thyme. Add the mushroom mixture to the chicken, and cook 10 minutes longer, until the chicken is tender. Add salt and pepper to taste.

PHASE 2

JERK CORNISH GAME HEN

"Jerk" is a Jamaican seasoning mixture that can be used for poultry, fish, and even to make a yogurt-based dip for vegetables. Usually fiery hot, this version is milder. It features two Microbiome Super-spices: turmeric, which fights inflammation and promotes digestive and brain health, and cinnamon, which helps to balance your blood sugar. You can also nourish your microbiome with onion and garlic while enjoying ginger's anti-inflammatory properties and its support for your digestive health.

1 SERVING

FOR THE JERK MIXTURE

   1 teaspoon chili powder

   ½ cup coarsely chopped onion

   3 garlic cloves, coarsely chopped

   1 tablespoon finely chopped fresh ginger

   2 teaspoons ground allspice

   1 teaspoon chopped thyme

½ teaspoon grated nutmeg

¼ teaspoon ground cinnamon

⅛ teaspoon ground clove

¼ teaspoon ground turmeric

¾ cup chopped fresh parsley

2 tablespoons olive oil

¼ cup fresh squeezed lime or lemon juice

2 tablespoons salt, or more to taste

1 teaspoon ground pepper

3 tablespoons water

FOR THE GAME HEN

1 Cornish game hen (1¼ to 1½ pounds)

½ tablespoon clarified butter

1. Combine all ingredients for the jerk mixture in a food processor and puree until smooth. Add more water if the paste is not pourable.

2. Preheat oven to 400°F.

3. Rub 1 tablespoon of the jerk seasoning in the cavity of the hen. Loosen the skin of the breast and legs of the hen, and spread 2 tablespoons of the seasoning on the flesh. Put the bird in a small roasting pan, and spread more seasoning on the skin. Top with the clarified butter.

4. Roast for 30 minutes or until the bird is golden brown and the juices run clear when the thigh is pierced with a fork. Let the hen "rest" for 3 minutes, and then serve. This dish is lovely with Mango Salsa (page 306).

PHASE 2

LAMB STEW PROVENCAL

Few combinations work better than a tangy orange, a crisp red wine, and the earthy meat of lamb. Herbs add fragrance and the Provencal aromas of southern France, while garlic, carrots, onions, and tomato help to heal your gut and nourish your microbiome. The chickpeas help women balance their hormones, especially during perimenopause and just after menopause.

You can make this stew in advance and keep it in the fridge for 3 or 4 days, or freeze it for several weeks. Serve with quinoa or brown rice.

2 SERVINGS

½ pound lamb, cut into 1-inch pieces

Salt and pepper

2 tablespoons olive oil

½ cup chopped onion

½ teaspoon chopped garlic

½ cup chopped carrots

1 cup cooked chickpeas

¾ cup diced tomatoes

½ cup red wine

1 cup Chicken or Beef Base (see pages 289 and 278)

1 teaspoon ground cumin

½ teaspoon dried tarragon

½ teaspoon dried thyme

½ teaspoon dried rosemary

1 teaspoon chopped orange zest

1 carrot, cut into ¼-inch rounds

Salt and pepper to taste

1 orange, peeled and sectioned

1. Sprinkle the lamb with salt and pepper. Sauté it in the oil in a small fireproof casserole over medium-high heat until browned, about 7 minutes. Add the onions and the remaining ingredients except for the salt, pepper, and the orange sections.

2. Bring the mixture to a boil, then lower the heat, and simmer on a low flame, covered, for an hour or until the lamb is tender but not falling apart. Add salt and pepper to taste. Garnish with orange sections.

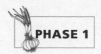

LEMON CHICKEN STEW

This piquant stew will really fill you up while incorporating three of our Microbiome Superfoods: onions, leeks, and garlic. Lemon and chicken is a wonderful flavor combination—something about the tangy lemon makes the chicken seem almost sweet.

You can cook this stew in advance and refrigerate it for up to 4 days or keep it frozen for several weeks. Reheat the defrosted stew in a 350°F oven until hot.

2 SERVINGS

1 pound chicken boneless, skinless breast or thighs

2 tablespoons olive oil, divided

⅓ cup chopped onion or leek

1 large carrot, peeled and cut into coins

1 parsnip, peeled and cut into coins

1 teaspoon freshly grated lemon zest

1 garlic clove, minced

⅓ cup fresh squeezed lemon juice

⅓ cup Chicken Base (page 289)

1 teaspoon chopped fresh rosemary

1 teaspoon chopped fresh thyme

Salt and pepper to taste

2 rosemary sprays (optional)

1. Preheat oven to 350°F.

2. In a sauté pan, lightly brown the chicken breasts in 1 tablespoon oil on medium-high heat for 10 minutes. Transfer the chicken to a baking pan.

3. Add remaining oil and onion until soft, about 3 minutes. Add the carrot and parsnip to the sauté pan, and cook for 5 minutes over medium-high heat until

lightly browned. Add the lemon zest, garlic, lemon juice, Chicken Base, chopped rosemary, and thyme, and cook for 5 minutes.

4. Pour the mixture over the chicken, and cover the baking pan with foil. Bake for 30 minutes until tender. Add salt and pepper to taste. Garnish with rosemary sprays, if desired.

The stew can be cooked up to 3 days in advance and can be frozen. Reheat in a 350°F oven until hot.

MEATBALLS WITH ROASTED SPAGHETTI SQUASH AND BASIL PESTO

 PHASE 1

Now you can enjoy spaghetti and meatballs, Microbiome Diet–style! The long, stringy noodle-like flesh of the squash makes a delicious gluten-free spaghetti that is loaded with nutrients to satisfy your taste buds while supporting your health. It also contains three Microbiome Superfoods—garlic, onions, and tomato.

To save you some cooking time, this recipe uses the extra frozen meatballs from the Sauerkraut and Meatball Soup on page 278. You can also cook the squash ahead of time, seed it, and shred it into "spaghetti." Then just reheat it when you're ready to make the dish.

2 SERVINGS

1 small spaghetti squash, pierced with the point of a
    knife in several places

½ onion, roughly chopped

2 tablespoons olive oil

1 garlic clove, minced

½ teaspoon oregano or marjoram

½ cup chopped roasted tomatoes

½ teaspoon salt

¼ teaspoon pepper

10 meatballs (see page 278)

3 tablespoons Basil Pesto (see page 282)

1. Preheat oven to 375°F. When heated, place the squash on a foil-lined sheet pan in the oven, and roast for 1 hour until soft. Let cool.

2. While the squash is roasting, sauté the onion in the olive oil over medium heat until soft, about 5 minutes. Add garlic and oregano. Lower the heat, and cook for 3 minutes; then add the tomatoes, salt, and pepper. Cook mixture for 5 minutes, then add the meatballs, and stew on low heat for 15 minutes. Cover and set aside.

3. When the squash is cool, remove the stem end, and cut in half lengthwise. Remove the seeds, and, with a fork, shred the squash into "spaghetti."

4. When ready to serve, mix the pesto into the squash in a saucepan, and heat for 6 minutes over medium heat.

5. Heat the meat balls and tomato sauce, heap it onto the spaghetti squash, and serve.

MEXICAN BEANS AND RICE WITH AVOCADO AND MANGO

PHASE 2

This exotic, tropically styled vegetarian stew is a wonderful study in contrasts: sweet mango and the fresh avocado setting off the warm, earthy rice and beans.

The recipe is for 6 servings because I think you will want to share it with guests—and you also get a lot of leftovers! Use the extra rice and beans in a salad with tomato and avocado. Or serve a smaller portion of the stew and salsa as a side dish with dinner entrées. The salsa will last for a week in an airtight container. Stored in its own airtight container, the stew will last two or three days.

Mango is loaded with digestive enzymes (see Chapter 4 for why that's important), and the avocado gives you healthy fats to support cell and brain health. The optional tomatillo is a small, green, tomato-like fruit often used in Mexican cooking. You can find it in either the produce section or the Latin foods section of your grocery store. It will add a little acid and texture to the salsa, which contrasts nicely with the sweet, smooth flesh of the mango.

6 SERVINGS

FOR THE BEANS

    1 cup dried black beans

    ½ cup chopped onion

    1 tablespoon ground cumin

    1 garlic clove, chopped

    1 tablespoon salt

1. Follow the recipe on the package if you want to presoak the beans. To cook the beans that day, put the beans in a pot and cover the beans with at least 3 inches of water. Place on high heat, bring to a boil, and immediately lower the heat to simmer. Simmer the beans for 10 minutes. Turn off the heat, and let the beans sit for 60 minutes.

2. Drain the liquid from the beans. Put in a clean pot and cover with 2 inches cold water. Put the heat on high, and bring to a boil. Add the onions, cumin, and garlic. Lower the heat to a simmer, and cook for 1 hour. Taste to see whether the beans are tender. Cooking time will vary depending on the age of the beans and the amount of absorbed water. Stir in salt.

FOR THE RICE

    ½ cup chopped onion

    1 tablespoon sunflower oil

    1 tablespoon coconut oil

    2½ cups brown rice

    1 13.5-ounce can organic coconut milk

    1½ cups water

    Salt and pepper to taste

1. Sauté the onion in the oils, and, when soft, add the rice. On low heat stir the rice until it becomes opaque. Add the coconut milk and water. At least 2 inches of liquid should cover the rice. Cover with a tight-fitting lid, and cook on low heat for about 30 minutes. Taste for tenderness. Salt and pepper to taste.

MANGO SALSA

    1 large ripe mango

    ¼ cup chopped onion

    1 small jalapeño pepper, seeded and rough chopped

1 small garlic clove, rough chopped

¼ cup chopped fresh mint

¼ cup chopped cilantro

3 tomatillos, grilled or charred in a cast-iron pan
(optional)

1 tablespoon fresh lime juice

Salt and pepper to taste

1. Combine all ingredients except for the salt and pepper in a blender, and pulse until almost smooth. Salt and pepper to taste.

THE TOPPINGS

1 ripe mango, cubed

½ cup diced jicama

1 ripe avocado, cubed

¼ cup chopped fresh cilantro

1. To serve, place beans on the rice, and top with the mango, jicama, avocado, and cilantro. Serve with the mango salsa and bowls of extra mango, avocado, jicama, and cilantro to pass around the table.

PHASE 2

Mussels Steamed in Beer

This dish is best made with Prince Edward Island mussels. Choose mussels that are closed so you know they are fresh. The serving size is for one because cooked mussels do not reheat well, but of course, you can multiply as needed for your dinner companions. This dish is best served with a warm, crusty, gluten-free bread that you can dip into the delicious beer broth, plus a simple green salad with Lemon Vinaigrette (page 263) or Citrus Vinaigrette (page 261).

Serves 1

1 pound mussels in shells

1 tablespoon olive oil

4 full sprigs of thyme

2 garlic cloves, minced

1 large shallot, chopped

½ teaspoon Dijon mustard

Salt and pepper

1 tablespoon chopped fresh tarragon

½ cup gluten-free beer

1. Rinse mussels under cold running water. Tap to close any mussels that are a little bit open. Discard any mussels that are broken, are wide open, or remain open after you tap them. Wash the shells, and "debeard" them by pulling off hairy clumps with your fingers.

2. Heat olive oil over medium heat in a soup pot with a tight-fitting lid. Add thyme, garlic, shallots, mustard, and a pinch of salt and pepper. Heat until shallots and garlic are softened, about 3 minutes. Add the tarragon, pour in beer, and bring to a simmer for about another 3 minutes. Add mussels, and cover the pot. Steam the mussels until they open, which usually takes 5 to 10 minutes. Discard any mussels that have not opened.

PAN-ROASTED COD WITH ORANGE CUMIN VINAIGRETTE

PHASE 1

Pan roasting is a simple, fast method for cooking many different types of fish. It's easy to get the hang of this approach, which allows you to have a nourishing dinner on the table within a few minutes. This particular recipe relies on cod, a mild, white, firm fish whose flavor is enhanced by a tangy, sweet orange cumin vinaigrette. Make some extra vinaigrette, and save it for a delicious salad dressing.

This dish goes great with Easy Sautéed Greens (page 294). The side dish brings in the Microbiome Superfood, garlic, as well as provide you with stress-reducing and brain-supporting B vitamins from the green leafy vegetables. Olive oil and flaxseed oil in the vinaigrette add healthy fats to promote cell and brain health.

1 SERVING

7 ounces cod filet

Salt and pepper

2 teaspoons clarified butter or 1 teaspoon olive oil
    and 1 teaspoon butter

1. Heat the oven to 425°F.

2. Salt and pepper the fish.

3. Heat on high heat a heavy-bottomed skillet or a cast-iron pan that is a little larger than the fish portion. When the pan is hot, add the butter. Add the fish top side down. Cook on high until the edges turn brown and the sides of the fish start to turn opaque, about 2 or 3 minutes. Do not turn the fish.

4. Put the pan in the oven, and cook at 425°F for about 6 to 8 minutes until the fish flesh is completely opaque and there is a crust on the bottom.

5. Turn the fish onto a plate by inserting the spatula under the end side of the filet. Serve with the vinaigrette (below) and Easy Sautéed Greens.

ORANGE CUMIN VINAIGRETTE

1½ teaspoons Dijon mustard

¼ cup freshly squeezed orange juice

⅛ cup cider vinegar

⅓ cup olive oil

1 tablespoon flaxseed oil

1 teaspoon chopped orange zest

1 teaspoon cumin

¼ teaspoon salt

¼ pepper

1. Whisk the mustard with the orange juice and vinegar. Add the oils, pouring in a slow stream. Add the zest, cumin, salt, and pepper.

2. Refrigerate the remainder for future use.

PAN-ROASTED SALMON

Wild-caught salmon has a high content of desirable Omega 3 fatty acids. Omega 3 molecules provide anti-inflammatory benefits as well as help to heal your gut walls, thereby improving your digestion and supporting your microbiome.

Please don't purchase farm-raised salmon. Find wild caught—it's far cleaner and way more nutritious.

I've had you pan-roast the salmon because it's a quick way to cook fish that produces enhanced flavor. Enjoy!

1 SERVING

Salt and pepper

7 ounces salmon filet or any thick fish

2 teaspoons clarified butter or 1 teaspoon olive oil and
 1 teaspoon butter

Lemon wedge

1 teaspoon melted butter with a sprinkling of tarragon
 (optional)

1. Heat the oven to 450°F. Place on high heat a heavy-bottomed ovenproof skillet or cast-iron pan that is a little larger than the fish portion.

2. Salt and pepper the fish.

3. When the pan is hot add the butter. Place the fish in flesh side down. Cook on high heat until the edges brown and an opacity starts to creep up the side of the fish, about 3 minutes. Do not turn the fish.

4. Put the pan in the oven. Cook for about 7 minutes, or until the fish flesh is opaque, firm, and there is a nice crust on the bottom. Then turn the fish onto a plate by inserting the spatula under the end side of the filet.

5. Serve with lemon wedge and tarragon butter, if desired.

STEAMED QUINOA

Quinoa looks like a grain, but the part you eat is actually the seeds. Protein-rich, filling, and full of antioxidants, quinoa is a great addition to any meal when you want a healthy choice to satisfy your craving for carbs. Quinoa is considered an anti-inflammatory food that also has significant antioxidant properties, but you won't be thinking about the health benefits when you're focused on the delicious taste. This buttery treat makes a great accompaniment to any meat or fish.

1 SERVING

1 teaspoon clarified butter or ghee

¼ cup rinsed and drained quinoa

½ cup water or Chicken Base

1 teaspoon chopped parsley

½ teaspoon chopped thyme (optional)

⅛ teaspoon salt

Salt and pepper to taste

1. Melt butter in a small saucepan over medium-low heat. Add the quinoa, and toast, stirring, for about 2 minutes. Add the water, and cook over low heat for about 8 minutes, until tender. Add the parsley, thyme, and salt. Add pepper and additional salt to taste.

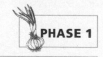

PHASE 1

TRADITIONAL CHICKEN SOUP

This protein-rich and healing chicken soup is based on a traditional "Grandma's Friday-night chicken soup" and makes a satisfying lunch or snack. Its warmth is good for your digestive tract, and the bones in the chicken soup base are full of key nutrients. Add extra vegetables if you like or, in Phase 2, add in some brown rice to make a filling and substantial dinner. Either way, the carrots, garlic, and onions in this soup and in the base are Microbiome Superfoods.

2 SERVINGS

2 cups Chicken Base (see page 289)

1 small carrot, peeled and sliced

1 parsnip, peeled and sliced

½ cup cut-up cooked chicken, or more

¼ cup snipped, rinsed dill

2 tablespoons fresh chopped parsley

Salt and pepper

1. Heat Chicken Base on low heat in a 6- or 7-inch saucepan for 5 minutes. Add carrot and parsnip, and cook over medium heat for 8 to 10 minutes, until tender. Add the cooked chicken. When the chicken is hot, after about 4 minutes, add the dill and parsley. Salt and pepper to taste.

2. Leftover soup may be frozen.

SEARED SCALLOPS

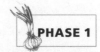 **PHASE 1**

Quick, easy, and delicious! This is the perfect meal to make when you want something that tastes fabulous and takes just a few minutes to cook. Be sure to buy "dry" scallops as opposed to "wet" ones. Wet scallops are treated with phosphates, a preservative that absorbs water. You can identify them because they are snow white. Dry scallops are natural and don't shrink when cooked—look for their natural cream color. You can ask your fishmonger to be extra sure. You might notice that large scallops are labeled "U10," a designation that means there are less than ten scallops to a pound.

2 SERVINGS

½ pound large dry sea scallops, preferably U10s

Salt and pepper

1 teaspoon olive oil

2 teaspoons clarified butter, divided

1 teaspoon lemon juice

1 teaspoon chopped parsley

1 teaspoon chopped chive

1 teaspoon chopped tarragon

1. Wash and dry the scallops. Sprinkle with salt and pepper.

2. Heat olive oil and 1 teaspoon butter in a heavy pan over high heat until almost smoking. Sear the scallops 1½ to 2 minutes on each side until a golden crust forms. Remove from heat.

3. Quickly melt remaining 1 teaspoon butter in the pan, add the lemon juice; cook for 1 minute over medium heat, then add the parsley, chive, and tarragon.

4. Pour the hot herb butter over the scallops, and serve immediately.

SNACKS

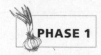

CURRIED ROASTED CAULIFLOWER

PHASE 1

This recipe is an addictive snack that can be eaten solo, added to a salad, or used as the side vegetable to a dinner entrée. The recipe includes turmeric, a ground spice that in India and Asia is used to promote health and has a history of medicinal uses in many cultures. And no wonder: this Microbiome Superspice helps heal inflammation, support your immune system, and promote brain and immune function. Onions and garlic add two more Microbiome Superfoods to the healthy mix.

This is a snack that will leave you feeling refreshed and satisfied, with no sugar rush or salt overload. Give it a try and see for yourself. (And if you need help buying or cooking with the fresh ginger, see the Mango Smoothie recipe on page 254 for instructions.)

4 SERVINGS

1 teaspoon minced garlic

2 tablespoons coconut oil

1 tablespoon olive oil

2 tablespoons chopped onion

2 tablespoons chopped fresh ginger root

1 cup coconut milk

1 large head cauliflower, trimmed and broken in to
   bite-size florets

1 tablespoon curry powder

¼ teaspoon turmeric

¼ teaspoon ground cumin

¼ teaspoon ground cardamom

¼ teaspoon mustard seeds (optional)

1. Preheat the oven to 400°F. Line a 13 x 18-inch sheet pan with parchment paper.

2. Warm the garlic in the oils in a medium saucepan over low heat, and add the onion and ginger. Sauté over low heat until the onion is soft, about 7 minutes. Add the coconut milk, and gently simmer for 5 minutes. Add the cauliflower, curry, turmeric, cumin, cardamom, and mustard seeds, if desired, and cook for 15 minutes, frequently ladling the coconut liquid over the cauliflower. The liquid will reduce substantially.

3. Transfer the cauliflower to the parchment-lined pan, and spoon the coconut milk mixture over the florets. Bake for 30 minutes until golden. Serve warm or at room temperature.

GAZPACHO SMOOTHIE

This afternoon tonic is a liquefied version of the popular cold Spanish soup. It is spicy, tangy, refreshing, and loaded with prebiotics from the chopped tomato and garlic. Olive oil and flaxseed oil give you some healthy fats, which are crucial for cell and, especially, brain health, while the protein powder gives you that midday energy boost to keep you functioning at optimal levels. Poured into a thermos, this smoothie is an easily portable snack or lunch. Shake vigorously before drinking.

1 SERVING

½ cup chopped tomato

½ cup chopped cucumber

2 heaping tablespoons chopped green pepper

1 teaspoon fresh lemon juice

½ cup water

2 tablespoons pea protein powder

¼ cup avocado

½ teaspoon ground cumin

1 tablespoon vinegar

1 teaspoon olive oil

1 teaspoon flaxseed oil

¼ teaspoon minced garlic

1 teaspoon salt

½ teaspoon jalapeño pepper, finely chopped, or
   ½ teaspoon hot sauce

3 ice cubes

1. Place all ingredients in a blender, and process until smooth.

OVEN-ROASTED KALE CHIPS

This addictive snack is also a superhealthy treat—a great way to load up on kale, which is one of the world's healthiest foods. Kale is rich in fiber, which is terrific for weight loss, and contains significant amounts of vitamins A, C, B6, and K as well as manganese and copper, providing you with antioxidant and anti-inflammatory protection and protection against cancer.

½ bunch kale leaves

1 tablespoon olive oil

Salt to taste

1. Preheat oven to 350°F. Line a large sheet pan with parchment paper.

2. Wash and thoroughly dry the leaves; wet leaves will make soggy chips. Remove the ribs from the kale leaves, and discard. Rip the kale into 1-inch pieces.

3. Rub the oil into the kale pieces; the leaves should be shiny but not oily. Sprinkle on salt.

4. Place the kale on parchment paper, and bake at 350°F for 10 minutes, or until crispy. Add more salt to taste, if desired.

ROASTED ASPARAGUS WITH LEMON

Asparagus helps improve digestive health, fights inflammation, and nourishes your microbiome, making it a natural prebiotic. But don't just choose asparagus for its health benefits—eat it because it tastes so good! Roasting this green vegetable enhances the flavor and makes it crunchy, while a splash of lemon makes it tangy. This recipe makes a nice big portion, so you can take some to work for a late-afternoon snack, dress some with Lemon Vinaigrette (page 263) for a flavorful salad, and reheat some to serve hot as a quick and easy side vegetable.

4 SERVINGS

24 large asparagus spears (about 2 pounds), with the
    hard round ends cut off

3 tablespoons olive oil

Kosher salt or coarse sea salt

2 tablespoons freshly squeezed lemon juice

Lemon slices

1. Preheat oven to 400°F. Oil a 13 x 18-inch sheet pan.

2. Place asparagus on an oiled sheet pan, and brush with oil. Sprinkle with salt.

3. Roast for 10 minutes, or until tender when pierced with a fork.

4. Sprinkle with lemon juice, and garnish with lemon slices. Serve either hot or cold.

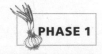

ROASTED SWEET POTATO CHIPS

You don't have to miss potato chips on the Microbiome Diet—you can satisfy your cravings with this crispy roasted savory-sweet snack. Use either sweet potatoes or yams, both of which are rich in antioxidants, dietary fiber, vitamins, and nutrients.

Slice the potatoes with a sharp knife, or invest $10 in a mandolin, a cutting device with different types of blades. Get one with a safety guard at your grocery store, at a housewares store, or online. They're great for all sorts of cutting and slicing; they save time and leave your veggies looking restaurant-beautiful.

1 TO 2 SERVINGS

1 large sweet potato
1 tablespoon olive oil
Salt to taste

1. Preheat oven to 300°F.

2. Scrub the sweet potato. Slice in thin, uniform slices.

3. In a bowl, toss the slices with the oil, and sprinkle with salt. Place on a single layer on cookie sheets, and bake for 1 hour, flipping every 15 minutes for even baking. When the slices begin to darken, watch carefully so they don't turn brown. The slices are ready when they are golden brown and crispy. The centers will be less crisp than the edges.

4. Salt to taste, and serve immediately. Leftovers, if there are any, will keep for 1 day. To reheat, crisp in the oven.

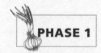

SPICED ROASTED CHICKPEAS

This addictive snack from Trinidad will last for days. Chickpeas, also called garbanzo beans, boost intestinal health and, as a fiber-rich food, provide a feeling of fullness. They also help women with hormonal balance, especially during perimenopause and right after menopause. The spice mixture includes turmeric, a Microbiome Superspice used in Indian and Asian cuisine with a history of medicinal benefits. Modern science tells us turmeric is a terrific anti-inflammatory that will boost your immune system and help heal your gut.

ABOUT 3 SERVINGS

1 teaspoon cumin
¼ teaspoon cayenne pepper
1 teaspoon curry powder
¼ teaspoon turmeric

1 teaspoon allspice

½ teaspoon cinnamon

¼ teaspoon fresh ground nutmeg

⅛ teaspoon ground cloves

1 teaspoon ground coriander

½ teaspoon chili powder, or more to taste

2 16-ounce cans organic chickpeas

1½ tablespoons olive oil

2 teaspoons kosher salt

Salt and pepper to taste

1. Preheat oven to 375°F.

2. Combine all spices (cumin through chili powder). Any remaining mixture can be stored and used as a rub for meat and poultry.

3. Drain the chickpeas, and rinse.

4. In a bowl, combine the chickpeas with the oil. Add 2 tablespoons of the spice mixture with the salt.

5. Spread the peas in one layer on a cookie sheet or shallow roasting pan. Place in oven, and bake until golden and crisp, about 30 to 40 minutes. Let cool to room temperature. Add more salt and pepper to taste if desired. Serve.

6. The spiced chickpeas can be stored in an airtight container. If they become soggy, rebake until crisp.

STEAMED ARTICHOKE WITH LEMON MUSTARD DIP

PHASE 1

Steamed artichoke is an unusual snack that can be made ahead of time. It takes a long time to eat, so it's great if you're feeling hungry because by the time you're done eating, you're full! Steamed artichokes also make a great side dish with a lunch salad.

There are lots of great health benefits associated with artichokes. They are powerful antioxidants that contain lots of nutrients as well as dietary fiber, which feeds your microbiome while making you feel full.

To eat the steamed artichoke, pull off a single leaf, dip it in the butter-lemon-mustard mixture, and slide the inside surface of the leaf over your bottom teeth to remove the flesh. Then throw the leaf away and pluck another. When you come to the fuzzy inner part—the choke, which covers the heart—just scrape it out with a spoon and throw it away. Then cut the heart and stem into bite-size pieces, dip each one into the sauce, and enjoy! I like to think of the delicious heart as the prize you get for working your way through the artichoke. Mmmm!

By the way, I'm having you make two artichokes and lots of extra dip so you can refrigerate both and reuse them the next time you make artichokes on your meal plans.

2 SERVINGS (2 ARTICHOKES)

2 medium artichokes
1 cup or more water
½ teaspoon lemon juice

For the artichoke

1. With scissors, cut off the thorns of the artichokes, leaving about an inch of stem. Place the artichokes in a steamer basket in a pot, and add water and lemon juice until it reaches the bottom of the steamer. Put a lid on the pot, and bring to a boil. Lower the heat to medium, and steam for approximately 40 minutes. To test for doneness, pierce the stem with a sharp knife. Let cool.

FOR THE DIP (6 servings)
6 tablespoons freshly squeezed lemon juice
3 teaspoons finely chopped lemon zest
1½ teaspoons Dijon mustard
1 teaspoon sea salt
9 tablespoons olive oil
3 teaspoons flaxseed oil
Salt and pepper to taste

1. Place all the dip ingredients in a small nonreactive bowl, and whisk. Add salt and pepper to taste.
2. Serve as a dip with a cooled artichoke. Refrigerate the leftover dip for future use.

STUFFED MUSHROOMS

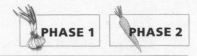

PHASE 1   PHASE 2

Two stuffed mushrooms make a satisfying hot snack. Or serve four stuffed mushrooms with Easy Sautéed Greens (page 294) for lunch. This recipe makes enough for one snack serving and one lunch entrée (with the Sautéed Greens). The garlic nourishes your microbiome, while the kale loads you up with iron and vitamin B to help you power through stress, promote brain function, and balance your hormones. In Phase 2 some sheep's milk or goat's milk cheese grated on top adds another texture and a salty kick.

1 LUNCH-SIZE SERVING
PLUS 1 SNACK-SIZE SERVING

2 tablespoons olive oil, divided

½ cup finely chopped onions

7 large white button or cremini mushrooms

2 cups kale, spines removed, rolled and thinly sliced

1 teaspoon minced garlic

½ teaspoon cumin

½ teaspoon salt

¼ teaspoon ground red pepper

Salt and pepper to taste

2 tablespoons grated sheep's milk cheese, optional
   in Phase 2

1. Preheat oven to 375°F.

2. Add 1 tablespoon oil to a medium sauté pan, and sauté the onions over medium-low heat, about 5 minutes, until tender.

3. Cut the stems off 6 mushrooms. Chop the last mushroom, and add to the onions; sauté for 2 minutes. Add the kale, garlic, cumin, salt, and red pepper, and cook on low heat until the mixture is soft, about 6 minutes. Add more salt and pepper to taste. Remove from heat.

4. Lightly brush the stemmed mushrooms with 1 tablespoon olive oil and stuff the mushrooms with the onion mixture. Place on a baking sheet, and bake for about 25 minutes, until the mushrooms are tender and the filling is heated through and golden. In Phase 2, top with grated sheep's milk cheese, if desired.

VEGETABLES WITH TURKISH GARLIC YOGURT DIP

PHASE 2

Yogurt with garlic and salt is a classic Turkish combination that brings out the flavor of vegetables. In this version garlic, onion, radish, and jicama give you the benefits of three Microbiome Superfoods.

You can make lots of extra dip, which refrigerates well for future use. Then experiment with different combinations of vegetables. Serving the dip over grilled eggplant is one delicious choice. Mixing it with sliced cucumbers for a cucumber salad is another. Whichever way you go, you are getting protein, probiotics, and a tart and tangy snack, the strong flavors of which leave you feeling satisfied both "stomach-wise" and "mouth-wise."

2 SERVINGS

1 teaspoon minced garlic

½ teaspoon sunflower oil or olive oil

½ teaspoon salt

1½ cups goat's or sheep's milk yogurt

Salt and pepper

1 tablespoon finely chopped fresh mint

½ cucumber, peeled, seeded, and cut into sticks

4 radishes, trimmed and halved

4 cherry tomatoes

¼ jicama, cut into sticks

6 endive leaves

1. In a small pan over low heat, warm the garlic in oil for about 2 minutes. Do not allow to brown. Drain the garlic into a small bowl, and mix with the salt. Add the yogurt, mixing well. Add salt and pepper to taste.

2. Put in a dipping bowl and sprinkle with fresh mint. Serve with raw vegetables.

METRIC CONVERSIONS

- The recipes in this book have not been tested with metric measurements, so some variations might occur.
- Remember that the weight of dry ingredients varies according to the volume or density factor: 1 cup of flour weighs far less than 1 cup of sugar, and 1 tablespoon doesn't necessarily hold 3 teaspoons.

— General Formulas for Metric Conversion

Ounces to grams	⇒ ounces × 28.35 = grams
Grams to ounces	⇒ grams × 0.035 = ounces
Pounds to grams	⇒ pounds × 453.5 = grams
Pounds to kilograms	⇒ pounds × 0.45 = kilograms
Cups to liters	⇒ cups × 0.24 = liters
Fahrenheit to Celsius	⇒ (°F − 32) × 5 ÷ 9 = °C
Celsius to Fahrenheit	⇒ (°C × 9) ÷ 5 + 32 = °F

— Linear Measurements

½ inch = 1½ cm
1 inch = 2½ cm
6 inches = 15 cm
8 inches = 20 cm
10 inches = 25 cm
12 inches = 30 cm
20 inches = 50 cm

— Volume (Dry) Measurements

¼ teaspoon = 1 milliliter
½ teaspoon = 2 milliliters
¾ teaspoon = 4 milliliters
1 teaspoon = 5 milliliters
1 tablespoon = 15 milliliters
¼ cup = 59 milliliters
⅓ cup = 79 milliliters
½ cup = 118 milliliters
⅔ cup = 158 milliliters
¾ cup = 177 milliliters
1 cup = 225 milliliters
4 cups or 1 quart = 1 liter
½ gallon = 2 liters
1 gallon = 4 liters

— Volume (Liquid) Measurements

1 teaspoon = ⅙ fluid ounce = 5 milliliters
1 tablespoon = ½ fluid ounce = 15 milliliters
2 tablespoons = 1 fluid ounce = 30 milliliters
¼ cup = 2 fluid ounces = 60 milliliters
⅓ cup = 2⅔ fluid ounces = 79 milliliters
½ cup = 4 fluid ounces = 118 milliliters
1 cup or ½ pint = 8 fluid ounces = 250 milliliters
2 cups or 1 pint = 16 fluid ounces = 500 milliliters
4 cups or 1 quart = 32 fluid ounces = 1,000 milliliters
1 gallon = 4 liters

— Oven Temperature Equivalents, Fahrenheit (F) and Celsius (C)

100°F = 38°C
200°F = 95°C
250°F = 120°C
300°F = 150°C
350°F = 180°C
400°F = 205°C
450°F = 230°C

— Weight (Mass) Measurements

1 ounce = 30 grams
2 ounces = 55 grams
3 ounces = 85 grams
4 ounces = ¼ pound = 125 grams
8 ounces = ½ pound = 240 grams
12 ounces = ¾ pound = 375 grams
16 ounces = 1 pound = 454 grams

ACKNOWLEDGMENTS

I WANT TO THANK MY AGENT, JANIS VALLELY, FOR HER HEARTFELT CARING FOR me and the Microbiome project. It was her keen ability to sense new and life-changing ideas that opened the gates for the publication of this book. Her belief in a down-to-earth, visceral approach to communication helped transform my approach to the writing of this book and to writing in general.

I also want to thank Rachel Kranz, without whom this book would never have come to fruition. Her great writing ability is only surpassed by her uncanny ability to be able to so swiftly download my ideas and so masterfully encapsulate them into words that shine. It is such a great privilege to work together with her on this project and others to come, for she shares my passion to see deeper, beyond the surface and the status quo, where the dots begin to come together and a new reality emerges.

I want to thank my marketing team leader Dee Dee DeBartlo. She not only quickly grasped the diverse ideas and messages of this book and my philosophy of healing in general and put it into simple words but also so quickly grasped the feeling and soul from where these ideas come. Working together, she and her associate, Jillian Sanders, make an insightful, knowledgeable, and powerful team.

I want to thank the brilliant art and website team leader Alexej Steinhardt of Roundhex and his wonderful studio manager, Tina Rath. As soon as I met them I just knew that they "get it."

I am so grateful to Renee Sedliar and the publishing team at Da Capo Press for publishing *The Microbiome Diet*. Renee had the foresight to realize that the microbiome diet represents a critical development in the chain of diet books and in health generally. Her critical edits brought the book to a new level. I also want to thank Amber Morris, my project editor at Da Capo, for so capably steering this book through all the twists and turns of production, and copy editor Josephine Mariea for her fine editing job. Thanks as well to Kate Burke, the associate director of publicity at Da Capo, whose efforts helped bring my book into the public eye. It is a pleasure to work with all of you, and I hope we will work together on many more books to come.

I want to thank Carole Clark, the chef who worked so hard on this project. She was so flexible and accommodating—a true team player. Carole made the microbiome diet approach to eating and cooking accessible to everyone. As you will see (and taste), she produced one masterpiece after another.

I can't thank enough my beloved teacher of blessed memory, Rabbi Brandwein. He taught me the great wisdom of Kabbalah that truly informs and directs the natural world, and I have come to learn that the knowledge of true Kabbalah also gives me a bird's-eye view of science. Just as Newton's Laws were influenced by this deep wisdom, my entire approach to medicine and healing and many of the ideas of this book emerge out of the fabric of the Kabbalistic worldview.

I want to thank my great friend Eliyahu Alfasi, who was also a student of Rabbi Brandwein and who has now become my teacher. He and I spent many hours discussing topics of this book, and he helped me articulate critical ideas. Who is better suited to be my teacher than the most knowledgeable person in the world on the Kabbalistic teachings of the greatest Kabbalist, Rabbi Ashlag, a man who truly lives by these lofty ideas? Who is more suited to be my teacher than someone who is also fluent in the great ideas of so many of the philosophers with whom Rabbi Ashlag was in dialogue? Thank you, Eliyahu.

Finally, I want to thank my beautiful wife, Chasya, who gave me the space and time to write this book. I want to express my deep gratitude to her for being the person I am not—someone who can oversee and manage big projects and keep me on track. Janis and Rachel, I am sure, are deeply thankful to her as well! Chasya all too often did double work in the house and with our children when I was so busy writing this book. Our life is one together, and therefore, she, in my mind, is the coauthor of this book.

RESOURCES

Betaine

Now, *www.nowfoods.com*. Their Betaine HCl is a very reliable source of hydrochloric acid.

Standard Process, *www.standardprocess.com*. Their product, Zypan, is a powerful combination of hydrochloric acid and digestive enzymes.

Thorne, *www.thorne.com*. Their Betaine HCl is a good source of hydrochloric acid for replacing stomach acid.

Enzymes

Integrative Therapeutics, *www.integrativetherapeutics.com*. Their product, Similase, soothes the gut and replaces needed enzymes.

Now, *www.nowfoods.com*. They make a very good product called Super Enzymes, which contain all the enzymes you need.

Microbiome Diet, *www.raphaelkellman.com*. My own brand of digestive enzymes, Replace, contains a very broad spectrum of powerful enzymes.

Orthomolecular, *www.orthomolecular.com*. Their product, Digest-zymes, contains a good, broad spectrum of digestive enzymes.

Fermented Foods

Bubbies, *www.bubbies.com*. Sauerkraut, kosher dill relish.

Bao Fermented Food and Drink, *www.baofoodanddrink.com*. Fermented and probiotic foods.

Immunotrion, *www.immunotrition.com*. Organic cultured vegetables of many types.

Pickle Planet, *www.pickleplanet.com*. Lacto-fermented foods.

Sunja's, *www.sunjaskimchi.com*. Kimchee of all types, from mild to spicy.

Wild Brine, *www.wildbrine.com*. All types of fermented foods.

Wise Choice Market, *www.wisechoicemarket.com*. Fermented foods.

Gluten-Free Foods

Against the Grain Gourmet, *www.againstthegraingourmet.com*

Bob's Red Mill, *www.bobsredmill.com*

Gluten Freeda Foods, *www.glutenfreedafoods.com*

Glutino, *www.glutino.com*

Udi's Gluten-Free, *www.udisglutenfree.com*

Grass-Fed Organic Meat, Poultry, and Eggs

Applegate Farms, *www.applegatefarms.com*

Organic Valley, *www.organicvalley.com*

Grow and Behold, *www.growandbehold.com*. For kosher as well as organic, free-range, and humanely treated animals.

Horizon Organic, *www.horizonorganic.com*

Pete and Gerry's Organic Eggs, *www.peteandgerrys.com*

Stonyfield Farm, *www.stonyfield.com*

Gut-Healing Products

Designs for Health, *www.designsforhealth.com*. Their product, GI Revive, is a powerful gut-healing compound that contains glutamine and gamma-oryzanol, which stimulates tissue repair, supports the synthesis of growth hormone, and may reduce body fat. I use this product frequently.

Metagenics, *www.metagenics.com*. Their product, Glutagenics, contains a high dose of glutamine, which helps heal gut walls.

Microbiome Diet, *www.raphaelkellman.com*. My own product, Repair, includes a wide range of nutrients to help heal the gut wall.

OrthoMolecular, *www.orthomolecular.com*. Their product, Inflammacore, contains glutamine and other healing compounds to repair the gut wall.

Organic Healthy Foods

EarthBound Farms, *www.earthboundfarms.com*
Diamond Organics, *www.diamondorganics.com*
Green for Good, *www.greenforgood.com*
Organics, *www.organics.com*
Organic Planet, *www.orgfood.com*
Shop Natural, *www.shopnatural.com*
Small Planet Foods, *www.cfarm.com*

Prebiotics

Ecological Formulas, *www.ecologicalformulas.com*. Their product, Cal-Mag Butyrate, is the one I prescribe to my patients.

Jarrow, *www.jarrow.com*. A source of inulin with FOS (fructooligosaccharides) for extra prebiotic support.

Klaire Labs, *www.klairelabs.com*. Their product, Biotagen, is a powerful combination of inulin and arabinogalactans that I often recommend to my own patients.

Now, *www.nowfoods.com*

Prebiotin, *www.prebiotin.com*

Standard Process, *www.standardprocess.com*

Xymogen, *www.xymogen.com*. Their product, ProBioMax Plus DF, is a powerful combination of arabinogalactans and probiotics that I often recommend to my own patients.

Probiotics

Organic3.com, *www.organic3.com*. A good source for *Lactobacillus gasseri*, which has been shown in studies to help with weight loss, as well as other probiotics. This company sells a probiotic powder that includes this vital bacteria.

Orthomolecular, *www.orthomolecular.com*. An excellent source for probiotics.

Microbiome Diet, *www.raphaelkellman.com*. My own personal line of probiotics.

Supersmart.Com, *www.supersmart.com*. A good source for *Lactobacillus gasseri*, which has been shown in studies to help with weight loss, as well as other probiotics. This company sells *Lactobacillus gasseri* as a separate capsule that you can take with your other probiotics.

Xymogen, *www.xymogen.com*. An excellent source for probiotics.

Products to Remove Unhealthy Bacteria

Designs for Health, *www.designsforhealth.com*. Their product, GI Microbe-X, is a powerful combination of herbs that will help balance your gut bacteria.

Metagenics, *www.metagenics.com*. Their product, Candibactin AR, will help eliminate unhealthy bacteria from your intestinal tract.

Microbiome Diet, *www.raphaelkellman.com*. My product, Remove, can be used as part of the Four Rs process. It contains a number of herbs that have a wide variety of antibacterial effects.

Protein Powder

Designs for Health, *www.designsforhealth.com*. This company's Pea Protein is a very reliable source of healthy protein.

Orthomolecular, *www.orthomolecular.com*. Core Restore is a protein powder I frequently recommend to my patients. It contains a potato-derived protein that seems to inhibit appetite.

Swedish Bitters

Standard Process, *www.standardprocess.com*. Their product, Digest, contains milk thistle, for liver support; dandelion root, a prebiotic; gentian; tangerine; and Swedish Bitters to stimulate the production of stomach acid.

Weight Loss Supplements

Douglas Labs, *www.douglaslabs.com*. Many of my patients have had good results with their product Metabolic Lean.

Life Extension, *www.lifeextension.com*. I often prescribe their Antiadipocyte Formula to my patients.

Xango, *www.xango.com*. Their Favao is an effective product.

NOTES

CHAPTER 1

10   "In 2008 the National Institutes of Health began a project to map the microbiome, triggering an enormous amount of exciting research." "Human Microbiome Project: Diversity of Human Microbes Greater Than Previously Predicted," *Science Daily*, May 21, 2010, www.sciencedaily.com/releases/2010/05/100520141214.htm.

11   "One of the first bacteria we encounter . . . allergy-related diseases, inflammatory bowel syndrome, and, again, obesity." Moises Velasquez-Manoff, "Are Happy Gut Bacteria Key to Weight Loss?" *Mother Jones*, April 22, 2013, www.motherjones.com/environment/2013/04/gut-microbiome-bacteria-weight-loss.

13   "According to some scientists . . . keeping the immune system in balance." Ibid.

13   "Martin J. Blaser, chair of the Department of Medicine . . . worldwide obesity epidemic." Michael Specter, "Exploring the Human Microbiome," *New Yorker*, October 22, 2012, www.newyorker.com/reporting/2012/10/22/121022fa_fact_specter.

13   "Other studies back up . . . other danger signs of metabolic disorder." E. Le Chatelier, et al., "Richness of Human Gut Microbiome

Correlates with Metabolic Markers," *Nature* 500, no. 7464 (August 29, 2013): 541–546, www.ncbi.nlm.nih.gov/pubmed/23985870.

15 "The results were startling . . . aren't really 'normal.'" Velasquez-Manoff, "Are Happy Gut Bacteria Key to Weight Loss?"

15 "As Velasquez-Manoff says ' . . . compared to a single page to-do list.'" Ibid.

19 "Yang-Xin Fu, MD, PhD . . . 'but also on the host's microbiome.'" Upadhyay, Vaibhav, et al., "Lymphotoxin Regulates Commensal Responses to Enable Diet-Induced Obesity," *Nature Immunology* 13, no. 10 (October 2012): 947–953, www.nature.com/ni/journal /v13/n10/abs/ni.2403.html.

20 "Consider this study by Walter Willett, MD . . . even when you consume more calories!" P. Greene, and W. Willet, "Pilot 12 Week Feeding Weight Loss Comparison: Low Fat vs. Low Carbohydrate Diets," Abstract 95, presented at the North American Association for the Study of Obesity's 2003 Annual Meeting.

22 "Researchers compared three groups of mice . . . perhaps by altering their microbiomes." A. P. Liou, M. Paziuk, J. M. Luevano Jr., S. Machineni, P. J. Turnbaugh, and L. M. Kaplan, "Conserved Shifts in the Gut Microbiota Due to Gastric Bypass Reduce Host Weight and Adiposity," *Science Translational Medicine* 5, no. 178 (March 2013): 178ra41, http://stm.sciencemag.org/content/5/178/178ra41.

24 "One group of researchers found that more than 80 percent of people . . . had initially lost." Gretchen Voss, "When You Lose Weight—and Gain It All Back," *Women's Health*, June 6, 10, www.nbcnews.com/id/36716808/ns/health-diet_and_nutrition/t /when-you-lose-weight-gain-it-all-back/.

24 "'Bad eating habits are not sufficient . . . metabolize the food we eat." Specter, "Exploring the Human Microbiome."

25 "A pioneering book . . . entitled *The Second Brain*." Michael D. Gershon, *The Second Brain: The Scientific Basis of Gut Instinct and a Groundbreaking New Understanding of Nervous Disorders of the Stomach and Intestines* (New York: HarperCollins, 1998).

28 "In January 2014 the *Proceedings* of the prestigious Mayo Clinic . . . on the microbiome into their clinical practice." Sahil Khanna, "A Clinician's Primer on the Role of the Microbiome in Human Health and Disease," *Mayo Clinic Proceedings* 89, no. 1 (January 2014): 107–114.

30   "Sarkis K. Mazmanian of the California Institute of Technology . . .
        'a fundamental part of us.'" Jennifer Ackerman, "The Ultimate So-
        cial Network," *Scientific American* 306, no. 6 (May 2012): 36–43.

CHAPTER 2

37   "NYU researcher Martin J. Blaser . . . average of every other year."
        Specter, "Exploring the Human Microbiome."
39   "Dr. Paresh Dandona . . . in a particularly dramatic way the inflam-
        matory role of diet." Velasquez-Manoff, "Are Happy Gut Bacteria
        Key to Weight Loss?"
41   "Groundbreaking research conducted by Patrice Cani at the Catho-
        lic University of Louvain in Brussels, Belgium . . . Good health and
        healthy weight are the result." Ibid.
46   "Feeding mice a probiotic apparently *blocked* weight gain. The probi-
        otic also helped decrease inflammation and improve the tight junc-
        tions in the epithelial walls." R. Mennigen, K. Nolte, E. Rijcken,
        M. Utech, B. Loeffler, N. Senninger, and M. Bruewer, "Probiotic
        Mixture VSL #3 Protects the Epithelial Barrier by Maintaining Tight
        Junction Protein Expression and Preventing Apoptosis in a Murine
        Model of Colitis," *American Journal of Physiology* 296, no. 5, pt. 1
        (2009): 1140–1149.
46   "Other studies have revealed that short-chain fatty acids block in-
        flammation in a variety of ways . . . and lower their triglycerides." Y.
        Furusawa, et al., "Commensal Microbe-Derived Butyrate Induces
        the Differentiation of Colonic Regulatory T cells," *Nature* 504, no.
        7480 (November 2013): 446–450; M. D. Säemann, et al., "Anti-
        Inflammatory Effects of Sodium Butyrate on Human Monocytes:
        Potent Inhibition of IL-12 and Up-Regulation of IL-10 Production,"
        FASEB Journal 14, no. 15 (December 2000): 2380–2382.
47   "In September 2013 . . . a high-fiber diet that was relatively low in
        unhealthy fats." V. K. Ridaura, et al. "Gut Microbiota from Twins
        Discordant for Obesity Modulate Metabolism in Mice," *Science*
        341, no. 6150 (September 6, 2013): 1079, www.sciencemag.org
        /content/341/6150/1241214.abstract.

CHAPTER 3

64   "In September 2013 . . . those other negative effects." A. N. Payne,
        C. Chassard, C. Lacroix, "Gut Microbial Adaptation to Dietary

Consumption of Fructose, Artificial Sweeteners and Sugar Alcohols: Implications for Host-Microbe Interactions Contributing to Obesity," *Obesity Reviews* 13, no. 9 (September 2012): 753–834.

66   "Researchers in Shanghai . . . more powerful than the 'slender' genes." N. Fei, and L. Zhao, "An Opportunistic Pathogen Isolated from the Gut of an Obese Human Causes Obesity in Germfree Mice," *ISME Journal* 7, no. 4 (April 2013): 880–884, www.nature .com/ismej/journal/v7/n4/full/ismej2012153a.html.

CHAPTER 5

75   "a December 2013 article published by the *Journal of the American Medical Association* . . . and other brain dysfunctions." Catherine Saint Louis, "Acid-Suppressing Drugs Linked to Vitamin B12 Deficiency, *New York Times* Blogs, December 10, 2013, *http:// well.blogs.nytimes.com/2013/12/10/acid-suppressing-drugs-linked -to-vitamin-b12-deficiency/*.

86   "The first incident . . . their cholesterol remained healthy." Robert Ornstein and Charles Swencionis, eds., *The Healing Brain: A Scientific Reader* (New York: Guilford Press, 1990), 88.

87   "The second 'experiment' . . . in this experiment." Robert M. Sapolsky, *Why Zebras Don't Get Ulcers: An Updated Guide to Stress, Stress-Related Diseases, and Coping*, 3rd ed. (New York: W. H. Freeman and Co., 2004).

CHAPTER 7

107 "So many studies . . . likely to lead to fat storage." K. A. Scott, et al., "Effects of Chronic Social Stress on Obesity," *Current Obesity Reports* 1, no. 1 (March 2012): 16–25, www.ncbi.nlm.nih.gov/pubmed /22943039.

108 "A 2010 study by a different team . . . gained more belly fat." S. J. Melhorn, E. G. Krause, K. A. Scott, M. R. Mooney, J. D. Johnson, S. C. Woods, and R. R. Sakai, "Meal Patterns and Hypothalamic NPY Expression During Chronic Social Stress and Recovery," *American Journal of Physiology: Regulatory, Integrative, and Comparative Physiology* 299, no. 3 (September 2010): R813–R822, www.ncbi .nlm.nih.gov/pmc/articles/PMC2944420/.

111 "in 2008 an Australian team . . . at the beginning of the semester." Simon R. Knowles, E. Nelson, and E. Palombo, "Investigating the

role of Perceived Stress on Bacterial Flora Activity and Salivary Cortisol Secretion: A Possible Mechanism Underlying Susceptibility to Illness," *Biological Psychology* 77, no. 2 (February 2008): 132–137, www.sciencedirect.com/science/article/pii/S0301051107001597.

113 "In fact, more than half of people . . . increased reactions to pain." Siri Carpenter, "That Gut Feeling," *American Psychological Association* 43, no. 8 (September 2012): 50, www.apa.org/monitor/2012/09 /gut-feeling.aspx.

114 "A 2010 experiment involved a Canadian team . . . and chronic fatigue syndrome." Mélanie G. Gareau, et al., "Bacterial Infection Causes Stress-Induced Memory Dysfunction in Mice," *Gut* 60, no. 3 (March 2011): 307–317, http://gut.bmj.com/content/early/2010 /10/21/gut.2009.202515.abstract.

114 "A 2011 experiment . . . feel less anxiety and depression." Carpenter, "That Gut Feeling."

114 "In 2013 a study from UCLA . . . improved ability to solve problems." K. Tillisch, et al., "Consumption of Fermented Milk Product with Probiotic Modulates Brain Activity," *Gastroenterology* 144, no. 7 (June 2013): 1394–1401.e4, www.gastrojournal.org/article /S0016–5085%2813%2900292–8/abstract.

CHAPTER 8

127 "A group of researchers at Swinburne . . . lowered cortisol levels." A. Scholey, C. Haskell, B. Robertson, D. Kennedy, A. Milne, and M. Wetherell, "Chewing Gum Alleviates Negative Mood and Reduces Cortisol During Acute Laboratory Psychological Stress," *Physiology & Behavior* 97, nos. 3–3 (June 2009): 304–312.

CHAPTER 10

154 "A 2004 study . . . the DNA of microbial bacteria." "Safety of Genetically Engineered Foods: Approaches to Assessing Unintended Health Effects," Committee on Identifying and Assessing Unintended Effects of Genetically Engineered Foods on Human Health, Institute of Medicine and National Research Council of the National Academies (Washington, DC: The National Academies Press, 2004).

155 "According to Dr. Jack Heinemann . . . 'genetically modified food.'" Jack Heinemann, "Report on Animals Exposed to GM Ingredients

in Animal Feed," Commerce Commission, New Zealand, November 24, 2009, www.biosafety-info.net/article.php?aid=645.

156   "Published by Emily Esfahani Smith . . . producing more inflammation." Emily Esfahani Smith, "Meaning Is Healthier Than Happiness," *The Atlantic*, August 1, 2013, www.theatlantic.com/health/archive/2013/08/meaning-is-healthier-than-happiness/278250/.

CHAPTER 11

168   "In June 2011 . . . the article noted." D. Mozaffarian, T. Hao, E. B. Rimm, W. C. Willett, F. B. Hu, "Changes in Diet and Lifestyle and Long-Term Weight Gain in Women and Men," *New England Journal of Medicine* 364 (June 23, 2011): 2392–2404, www.nejm.org/doi/full/10.1056/NEJMoa1014296?query=featured_home&.

168   "A year earlier . . . insulin sensitivity and inflammation." H. Sadrzadeh-Yeganeh, I. Elmadfa, A. Djazayery, M. Jalali, and M. Chamary, "The Effects of Probiotic and Conventional Yoghurt on Lipid Profile in Women," *British Journal of Nutrition* 103, no. 12 (June 2010): 1778–1783, http://journals.cambridge.org/action/displayAbstract?fromPage=online&aid=7807665.

170   "Inulin has also been shown . . . *British Journal of Nutrition*." Beatrice L. Pool-Zobel, "Inulin-Type Fructans and Reduction in Colon Cancer Risk: Review of Experimental and Human Data," *British Journal of Nutrition* 93, Suppl. S1 (April 2005): S73-S90, http://journals.cambridge.org/action/displayAbstract?fromPage=online&aid=922696.

INDEX